Realignments in the
Welfare State

Realignments in the Welfare State

HEALTH POLICY IN THE UNITED STATES, BRITAIN, AND CANADA

MARY RUGGIE

COLUMBIA UNIVERSITY PRESS

NEW YORK

Columbia University Press
Publishers Since 1893
New York   Chichester, West Sussex
Copyright © 1996 Columbia University Press
All rights reserved

Library of Congress Cataloging-in-Publication Data

Ruggie, Mary, 1945–
    Realignments in the welfare state : health policy in the United
States, Britain, and Canada / by Mary Ruggie.
       p.   cm.
    Includes bibliographical references and index.
    ISBN 0-231-10484-7 (cloth). — ISBN 0-231-10485-5 (paper)
    1. Medical policy—United States. 2. Medical policy—Canada.
3. Medical policy—Great Britain. 4. Welfare state. 5. Medical
care—Finance—Government policy—United States. 6. Medical care—
Finance—Government policy—Canada. 7. Medical care—Finance—
Government policy—Great Britain. I. Title.
    RA393.R84   1996
362.1—dc20

96-10966
CIP

∞

Casebound editions of Columbia University Press books are printed
on permanent and durable acid-free paper.
Printed in the United States of America
c 10 9 8 7 6 5 4 3 2 1

For John and Andreas,
always

Contents

Preface

The news from Washington in the fall of 1995 tests one's nerve in arguing that the welfare state is not being dismantled. As Congress is poised to increase recipient payments for Medicare, reduce its contribution to Medicaid, and fold Medicaid and other social welfare programs (such as Aid to Families with Dependent Children) into block grants, the retrenchment that seemed peculiar to the Reagan era has acquired a new and more encompassing force. Presidential vetoes may forestall these particular eventualities, but the drive for cost-driven reform will continue, not only in Washington but in London and Ottawa as well. This book does not offer solutions to the dilemmas confronting contemporary welfare states. Instead, it addresses a broader issue: Are we finally at the end of the welfare state? My answer remains no.

The welfare state as we have known it has been waning for some time. But its core persists. We have so come to focus on the word *state* and on its specification as ``central government expenditure'' that we have forgotten the fuller meaning of the welfare state: a collective commitment to improving individual life chances and social well-being. The role of the central government as chief financier and provider of social benefits is declining. Instead the state is beginning to adopt another role, one of prodding other actors to fill the gap left by changing state functions and ensuring that they do so without unduly jeopardizing accepted normative standards of equity in access and outcome. Moreover, as local public, quasi-public, and private-sector actors enter the arena of social provision, the state is not simply handing over the baton. It is actively negotiating agreements for service delivery, brokering liaisons among providers and between providers and recipients, and overseeing a complex network of social care. These new state activities can no longer be captured by quantitative terms that presume to measure the role of the state. In short, we are witnessing not a reduced role but a decidedly different one.

These changes are still in their formative stages and may yet falter. If they fail, we may see a return to an earlier era of welfare state organization, characterized by a clear boundary between the responsibilities and accountabilities of state and social actors. As we know from history, however, setbacks are episodic and demands for reform perennial. If successful, the changes discerned in this study could result in innovative welfare state structures and modalities.

Because this book has been so many years in the making, I have watched many ebbs and flows in health care policy and politics. It is my scholarly predilection to stand back from the fray and explore the big picture, identifying the enduring structural features within which policy choices are made. I argue that despite the empirical differences among the health care systems in the United States, Britain, and Canada, similarities can be found at a higher level of abstraction, which I operationalize as three types of state/society relations in health care policy developments. A segmented policy regime is based on the traditional division of authority and fundamental bifurcation of state and society characteristic of liberal welfare states. An interventionist policy regime occurs when governments attempt to correct market failures; in liberal welfare states such intervention is frequently deeper than intended, resulting in tensions in state/society relations. I suggest that both of these modes of social action may be yielding to an integrative policy regime based on collaborative interactions between state and social actors who construct a negotiated social order. In an integrative policy regime the role of the state appears to be reduced, but insofar as the state acts as the arbiter of last resort, its authority is firm. These distinctions help us understand how and why the present face of the welfare state is different from the past. The utility of my approach is that it proffers a vision of change and identifies forces conducive to change. Directions of change can only be imputed, especially when history is in the making.

Many people have helped me in the long and sometimes trying task of writing this book. Some entered my life and then left it again, because of my moves from Barnard College to the University of California, San Diego, and then back to Columbia University, or because my research trips spanned many changes in administrations and administrators. I find it impossible even to begin a list of acknowledgments for fear of missing someone. A few others have stayed in my life and consistently offered the encouragement and sustenance that comes only with true friendship and much love. I dedicate this book to two of them.

List of Acronyms

AALL   American Association for Labor Legislation
AAMC   American Association of Medical Colleges
AHA   Area Health Authority
AMA   American Medical Association
BMA   British Medical Association
BNA   British North America Act
CCF   Cooperative Commonwealth Federation
CCSC   Central Consultants and Specialists Committee
CHA   Canada Health Act
CHIA   Canadian Health Insurance Association
CHO   Community Health Organization
CLIA   Canadian Life Insurance Association
CMA   Canadian Medical Association
CON   Certificate of Need
DHA   District Health Authority
DHHS   Department of Health and Human Services
DHSS   Department of Health and Social Services
DRG   Diagnosis-Related Group
EPFA   Established Programs Financing Act

ERISA	Employee Retirement Income Security Act
FHSA	Family Health Services Agency
GAO	General Accounting Office
GDP	Gross Domestic Product
GNP	Gross National Product
GP	General Practitioner
HCFA	Health Care Financing Administration
HEW	(Department of) Health, Education, and Welfare
HIDS	Hospital Insurance and Diagnostic Services Act
HMO	Health Maintenance Organization
HSO	Health Service Organization
IPA	Independent Practice Association
MAAG	Medical Audit Advisory Group
NDP	New Democratic Party
NHS	National Health Service
OBRA	Omnibus Budget Reconciliation Act
OECD	Organization for Economic Cooperation and Development
OMA	Ontario Medical Association
PPO	Preferred Provider Organization
PPRC	Physician Payment Review Commission
PRO	Peer Review Organization
PSRO	Professional Standards Review Organization
RAWP	Resource Allocation Working Party
RHA	Regional Health Authority
TCMP	Trans-Canada Medical Plans
VPS	Volume Performance Standards

Realignments in the
Welfare State

Chapter One

The Welfare State:
Retrenchment, Stagnation, or Transformation?

The 1980s witnessed heated debates about the future of the welfare state. Critics were no longer content merely to warn that social expenditures must be curbed. They focused on active dismantling. By the early 1990s there was uncertainty about the condition of the welfare state. Because of retrenchment, further expansion of the welfare state was being curtailed. But at the same time, many of its functions continued to be performed. The mid-1990s saw renewed attacks on the welfare state, which were especially vociferous in the United States. But ambiguity about future directions persists. Some of the ambiguity stems from the term *welfare state* and the governmental role it implies. As we will see in this chapter, because of vast differences in what states are doing, there is no longer a commonly agreed-to definition of the welfare state. In general, governments remain actively involved in social provision, but they are acting less as providers themselves and more as overseers of broader-based social provision. This book explores the changing role of the state in one area of social policy: health care. And it does so in three countries—the United States, Britain, and Canada—whose welfare state systems were most vulnerable to dismantling in the 1980s but continue to provide fundamental social benefits in the 1990s. These three and many other welfare states have been experimenting with alternative forms of social provision. How these alternative forms signal both persistence and transformation of the welfare state is the central concern of this study.

The present chapter outlines the debate about the welfare state—its practical as well as its ideological dimensions. It shows that retrenchment, measured as reductions in the size and reach of the welfare state, has had mixed results, which are difficult to interpret conventionally. We have become so accustomed to thinking about the welfare state in terms of an expansion of state services that we cannot yet fully conceptualize new roles for both state and social actors in social provision. But new roles are emerging. The following review of the literature examines the shortcomings of prevailing conceptualizations and provides some insights on which to base alternative formulations. At the end of the chapter, I propose a typology for the analysis of health care—past, present, and future—as an instance of this evolution in the welfare state.

Retrenchment: Its Rise and Demise

With the elections of Margaret Thatcher, Ronald Reagan, and their counterparts in several other countries, all bent on subordinating the state to market discipline, the long-predicted crisis of the welfare state seemed to be at hand. Reports of declining expenditures on social provision, the elimination of social programs, increased user fees for social services, and experiments in privatization appeared in all the advanced industrial countries. Even in Scandinavia, which experienced a tax backlash in the 1970s, politicians began to use the vocabulary of retrenchment in the 1980s (Johansen 1986). As unemployment figures rose along with budget deficits and as public assistance fell ever shorter of meeting growing needs, there was a generalized sense that the tenuous "Keynesian consensus" that had sustained the expansion of the welfare state had come to an end (Quadagno 1987). One assessment, jarring when first voiced by a sympathetic observer, soon became commonplace: "the welfare state throughout the industrialised West is in disarray. . . . [Its] legitimacy is in serious doubt" (Mishra 1984, pp. xiii, xiv).

The immediate backdrop for this note of despair was the economic downturn that had begun in the 1970s. It had always been assumed that the welfare state expanded during periods of economic growth. But what about the reverse? Would not economic decline necessarily undermine the foundations of the welfare state and cause its erosion? Dissection of the links between the welfare state and the economy followed. Many studies concurred that the welfare state had reached its limits.

A Premortem

One of the early studies to substantiate the relationship between economic downturn and declining social spending was a 1981 OECD report on *The Welfare State in Crisis*. The report defined the crisis as a slowdown in the rate of increase in expenditures on social programs (including education, health, pension, unemployment compensation, income maintenance, and welfare services). It attributed the slowdown to the low-growth performance that economies began to experience after the first oil shock of 1973–1974. And it suggested that, in this economic climate, "some social policies (unemployment compensation, minimum wages and high payroll taxes) have negative effects on the economy . . ." (OECD 1981:5). The implication that social spending should be reduced to *relieve* the economy seized the attention of researchers and newly elected conservative governments alike. Studies began to document the adverse economic consequences of social expenditures, as well as the consequences of deteriorating economic conditions on the future of the welfare state. The OECD published a follow-up report in 1985 entitled *Social Expenditures*. It amply demonstrated that declining annual growth rates in GDP were accompanied by slower rates of growth in social expenditures. Governments, it seemed, were responding to economic imperatives. An era of retrenchment appeared to have set in for the welfare state.

Retrenchment in the welfare state was not only a response to economic facts of life, but also a reflection of growing discontent with the performance of the welfare state. The realization that expenditures had not reduced social inequalities was widespread and was not confined to the United States—where the skewed relationship between, for example, expenditures on education and basic literacy rates, health spending and infant mortality rates, welfare spending and poverty seemed to mock the very term *welfare state*. Even in the European social democracies, questions were raised about perverse correlations between improved working conditions and worker alienation (absenteeism despite ever-shorter work-weeks, production problems due to alcoholism). The welfare state stood charged as contributing to alienation among young people (high youth unemployment despite active labor market programs, out-of-wedlock births despite free contraceptive and abortion services) (Popenoe 1988). While there had always been ideological opposition to the welfare state, these sour notes were ringing louder and clearer. Something had gone wrong with the prevailing mode of realizing the ideals of the welfare state, if not with the very foundations of those ideals. What was behind this malaise?

Conservative scholars and politicians rose to the occasion in the 1980s to provide an answer. The conservative position that government's power of taxation is a limited transfer of authority that had been transgressed by overspending formed the basis for an indictment of welfare state activities. Glazer (1988:5) argued that government activism had created a spiral of deepening problems and doomed policies: "any policy has dynamic aspects such that it also expands the problem, changes the problem, generates further problems." Politicians were blamed for having promised more than government could reasonably deliver; liberalism was blamed for acting on the dictum that "for every problem there is a policy"; the bureaucracy was blamed for having bred civil servants who perpetuated the welfare state for their own careerist reasons.[1] Murray (1984) castigated the welfare state for worsening the distressing situation of millions of individuals and their families by depressing their incentive to work and condemning their spirit to dependence on government. The conservatives' formulation of the problem also contained clear remedies: Roll back the activities of government and free the private and voluntary sectors to (re-)assume their rightful place in the social, political, and economic order.

The simplicity of the conservatives' analysis and its apparent approximation to ongoing retrenchment had been anticipated, ironically, in earlier neo-Marxist treatises. The basic Marxist position on the crisis in the welfare state was first outlined by O'Connor (1973). Gough (1979:152) later stated the main point succinctly: "The welfare state is a product of the contradictory development of capitalist society and in turn it has generated new contradictions which every day become more apparent." Marxists hold that because of the contradictory nature of the state's accumulation and legitimation functions (accumulation requires investment and therefore constrains current expenditures; legitimation requires current expenditures and therefore constrains investment),[2] the contemporary welfare state is locked into a self-paralyzing dilemma. The state's attempts to satisfy particular and opposing interests require ever-increasing resources and expenditures. And insofar as its expenditures never adequately appease anyone, the state's ability to continue taxing and spending is impeded. The resulting fiscal crisis, most visible in the huge budget deficits of advanced capitalist welfare states, produces social anomie as well as economic and political stalemate (Habermas 1976).[3] In the end, Marxist thought leads us to conclude that the welfare state is doomed. Unlike conservatives, Marxists offer no visionary paths to salvation.

If two such opposed ways of thinking came to the same conclusion, was it safe to assume that they were both right? Or could they both be wrong?

The Welfare State Lives

Beginning in the mid-1980s, a new set of studies argued that the welfare state was not in crisis and had not collapsed. Researchers offered data showing that although the rate of increase in social expenditures had declined, the overall trend toward expansion was continuing, albeit moderately and unevenly. Indeed, some went so far as to claim that "provided economic growth is of the order of 1 per cent or more annually, there is no public expenditure crisis" (O'Higgins and Patterson 1985:129). Scholars who closely examined the components of welfare state policies and programs suggested that "it is misleading to talk of the unraveling or dismantling of the welfare state. Efforts at retrenchment have been more selective and far less successful than many observers apparently believe . . ." (Brown 1988:6). By the early 1990s, then, it seemed that the era of retrenchment had become an era of confusion.

Some researchers had maintained all along that the welfare state was not eroding and that the "Keynesian consensus" that was so important to welfare state growth continued to inform social expenditure decisions. For example, in a study of 23 OECD countries Schmidt (1983) found that during economic downturns, countries that are less successful economically tend to *increase* expenditures for unemployment benefits, social assistance, and early retirement schemes more than countries with more resilient economies. Reinforcing the tendency to increase expenditures are such political factors as dominance of social democratic parties and corporatist forms of wage compromise. Schmidt (1983:5–6) summarized his position thus: in the early 1970s, "public authorities were generally more inclined to contain setbacks to economic growth, to expand the scope of state-financed programmes, and to expand labour market policies and social security expenditures. [After the second oil price shock of the late 1970s, the] restrictive policy stance taken by the Reagan administration and the Thatcher government was the exception." This analysis suggested that the welfare state in the United States and Britain—where it has always been weak—might be in jeopardy, but the welfare state in general, especially where it is tied to a social democratic political order, lives on.

The OECD went even further. By 1987 another of its reports argued that, although it is true that "Social policies cannot afford to ignore any negative impacts that certain provisions may have on economic performance," the reverse also holds: "economic policies need to take account both of the social consequences and of the social objectives of economic change, and of the positive contribution which effective social protection can make to economic dynamism" (OECD 1987:7).

What Is the Welfare State?

When all is said and done, we cannot determine with any certainty whether the welfare state itself has survived into the 1990s or whether only some social programs have survived. Governments are adapting to economic constraints, but it is difficult to generalize about how they are adapting—what is being cut, what not, and what other changes are occurring in social provision.[4] How are we to understand the welfare state today?

For decades definitions of the welfare state rested on two dimensions—the commitment of the state to enhancing social equality and the use by the state of social expenditures to achieve that end. Both of these dimensions presupposed the expansion of state resources and outlays for social programs. Wedderburn's (1965:127) observation captures this classic understanding: there is "a central core of agreement that the welfare state implies a commitment of some degree which modifies the play of market forces in order to ensure a minimum real income." Hage and Hanneman's (1980:46) definition is simpler and more mechanical: A welfare state exists when "more than 10 percent of GNP is allocated to public expenditure on health, public assistance, and social insurance programs." These definitions are no longer adequate. An anomaly exists in the welfare state that needs clarification: At least some parts of the welfare state are surviving, but the *state* is not performing the same roles it once did.

A clear understanding of the present role of the state in the welfare state is hard to come by because most of our thinking is still embedded in the paradigm of steady expansion. Contrary to this view, government fiscal resources have become strained and government's role in expenditure-based social programs has therefore changed. Nevertheless, social provision continues, if not by government then by other social actors. Moreover, governments are overseeing this broader base of social provision. How can we clarify the role of the state to capture this new complexity of the welfare state? We must examine not only what the state itself is doing but also what the state is occasioning other social actors to do. And we must consider why other social actors, and not the state alone, may now be more involved in social provision. In sum, we must transcend dualistic thinking and conceptualize a new relationship between the state and society.

Social Relations in the Welfare State

The relationship between state and social actors in the welfare state is, in Weber's terms, associative (as opposed to communal): "the orientation of social action within [an associative relationship] rests on a rationally motivated adjustment of interests or similarly motivated agreement, whether the basis of rational judgment be absolute values or reasons of expediency" (Roth and Wittich, eds, 1978:40–41). To understand this associative relationship we need to investigate the various principles and norms that underpin it, as well as the social dynamics involved. The literature on the welfare state offers three basic conceptions of the roles and relations among state and social actors, which we can characterize as society-centric, state-centric, and interdependent.

In the first, the society-centric model, the state simply reacts to society's demands, either by acceding to dominant social groups or by attempting to hold off certain social demands. In this asymmetrical relationship the state is a secondary actor and its authority is "borrowed" from society. The most common version of the society-centric model is the "logic of industrialism" argument, which holds the functionalist position that industrialization creates social needs to which states respond with social spending.[5] Some scholars have expanded the position to argue that demographic imperatives now shape state behavior.[6] Pluralists also espouse a society-centric perspective, arguing that government decision making follows the demands of dominant interest groups.[7]

A second perspective, the state-centric view, reverses this hierarchy and envisions the state as intervening in the private affairs of society or the dynamics of the market, as in Wedderburn's definition. State actors claim a measure of authority over social actors and attempt to direct the activities of social actors accordingly. Since social actors commonly resist state efforts, a more adversarial social dynamic ensues between state and social actors than is depicted in the society-centric model.

The state-centric model has been supplemented in studies of the bureaucratic capacity of the state. Heclo (1974) focuses on the increasing centralization of state functions and the role of institutional learning in policy formation. Orloff and Skocpol (1984), among others, demonstrate how the timing and sequencing of democratization and bureaucratization account for differences in the appearance of certain benefit programs. In general, early democratization untamed by bureaucratization produced patronage-oriented welfare programs (as in the United States and Canada); countries where state bureaucratization preceded or accompanied democratization (Britain) developed more systematic welfare state policies and programs (Orloff 1993).

In addition, several students of the American welfare state explain both American exceptionalism and the nature of the American welfare state within a state-centric model. They argue that powerholders in the United States have not simply or consistently reacted to political and social demands, as pluralists hold. Some scholars (Quadagno 1982; Skocpol and Ikenberry 1983; Skocpol 1992) demonstrate that American welfare state development has been led by powerful political actors who are not averse to social progress. Skocpol maintains that the state comes to acquire its own capacity to weather demands and direct state resources toward collective goals: "states affect political and social processes through their policies and their patterned relationships with social groups" (1985:3).

A third perspective, an interdependence model, seeks to explore the possibility of various forms of accommodative, cooperative, or collaborative interactions between state and social actors that place them in a more mutually supportive relationship. Some students of comparative welfare states, particularly those who study certain European social democracies (such as Sweden) attempt to bridge the society-centric and state-centric models by emphasizing that the state consists, for example, of a strong labor constituency (Stephens 1979; Korpi 1983). In responding to labor demands social democratic governments actively strive to reduce social inequalities. To do so, government must have the authority to act as an agent of equality, which necessitates considerable state intervention. At the same time, the ability of the state to intervene rests on the active support of civil society.

The formulations of neopluralists as well as theorists of neocorporatism are particularly helpful in understanding interdependent roles and relations among state and social actors in contemporary welfare states. Neopluralist suggestions for relieving the over-centralized, overbureaucratized, and overloaded welfare state focus on a return to the authority of citizens as the driving force in decision making and policy implementation.[8] In addition, neopluralists call for decentralization of all levels of government. At the local level, decentralization includes citizen participation, so that, for example, decisions about provision flow from a partnership between social services staff and the recipients of services (Johnson 1987:59).

These prescriptions are of particular interest to an understanding of interdependence when applied to the commercial or for-profit private sector. Unlike conservatives, who would like to firm up the boundary between government and the private sector, neopluralists affirm the utility of mixed institutional forms (see Ostrander, Langton, Van Til, eds., 1987). Neopluralists appreciate that greater use of the private, for-profit, or market sector can not only improve social provision but even potentially foster increases in income equality (Rein 1989). They also hold that the various ways in which governments support privatization efforts can strengthen the ties between the two sectors and thereby lead to a social integration without undermining the integrity of the cooperating sectors. Neopluralists thus perceive a social welfare mix of some sort, one that involves state support for nonstate activities: "the state is not viewed any more as the centre but as a kind of moderator of a plurality of societal projects" (Evers 1990:25).[9]

Those neocorporatist theorists who are explicitly interested in changes in the welfare state critique both the pluralist and conservative as well as the orthodox Marxist versions of the crisis of the welfare state and the solutions offered.[10] Thus, neocorporatism offers a middle way not only between a command system and a pluralist model of welfare state development, but also between the conservative and the Marxist quests to dismantle the welfare state. Cawson (1982), for one, understands the crisis of the welfare state to be structural, pertaining specifically to the development of a dual economy consisting of a competitive market sector and a corporate sector, with the latter having become increasingly important. Moreover, the dual economy has spawned a dual state.[11] That is, because of the development of powerful corporate groups, the basis of policy-making in contemporary welfare states has changed from competitive politics to corporatist politics, characterized by a process of negotiation between the state and corporate groups. In corporate policy-making, neither the state nor the corporate group dominates. Each actor brings a measure of independent power to the negotiation process, and each accedes to the power of the other during the negotiations.[12]

Whereas for Cawson corporatism becomes a problem in the contemporary welfare state, signaling as it does the loss of democracy, for Mishra (1984) corporatism suggests a solution.[13] Mishra calls the corporatist form of a post-Keynesian, post-Beveridge construct an integrated welfare state.[14] For Mishra, integration rests on the fundamental coordination of social policy with the economy. That is, social policy is seen as advancing the cause of economic growth. Governments promote social policy as much as possible and to the extent that it helps the economy.[15] Social integration is an active force in Mishra's model, and the role of the state is systemic. Collaboration between major organized interests (primarily labor and business) requires that the state curtail "free-for-all pluralism." At the same time, the tripartite (state, business, labor) structure of decision making in a corporatist order bypasses and downgrades to some extent "the formal political order" of parliament and political parties (Mishra 1984:105).

By emphasizing the voluntary nature of corporatist participation and structures, Mishra (like Cawson) is attempting to depict an authoritative, but not authoritarian, state. However, he does not appreciate that while voluntarism may pertain to major organized interests, democratic governments cannot choose whether or not to interact with social actors—they must, in some fashion. Despite Mishra's efforts to conceptualize state autonomy, the role of the state he presents follows from the achievement or failure of the voluntarily reached agreements of major organized interests. Although he is depicting a state whose primary function is to integrate, its success in doing so, and thereby its ability to act authoritatively, depends on the prior success of collaboration between major organized interests. When that collaboration fails or falls short of the integrative goals of the state, the state is left either to impose its goals (as in authoritarianism) or to demur (as in pluralism).[16]

These reconceptualizations of the welfare state offered by neopluralists and neocorporatists are useful because they suggest changes in the activities of the welfare state—shifts from state provision to state facilitation, from state accumulation and expenditure of resources to state guidance in engaging other social actors to perform socially desirable tasks. Even though these studies do not offer a fully consistent framework for understanding interdependent roles and relations among state and social actors, their insights can be modified to understand the anomaly in the contemporary welfare state that I seek to resolve.

Liberal Welfare States: Variations on a Theme

Based on aggregations of various features of social policies and programs,[17] scholars have differentiated three broad types of welfare states, which correspond roughly to the three perspectives outlined earlier. In one, the liberal democratic type, the state defers to market forces for policy guidance. In another, the social democratic type, the state takes command of market forces and engages in more active redistribution of social resources than in the other two types. The characteristics of a third type of welfare state are unsystematic in the literature, except for the effort to identify forces that circumvent the dominance of both market and state. Because in many cases of this third type, the workplace serves as the locus of social benefits, it is commonly referred to as a corporatist type of welfare state. Corporatist welfare states vary in the extent to which either the market or the state is involved in the allocation, quantity, and quality of social benefits. Where countries are placed in these typologies may vary, depending on which countries and which policies are being compared, and what point the author wishes to emphasize. Thus, typologies are best considered as heuristic devices.

Without belittling the significant differences among them, the United States, Britain, and Canada typically belong to the type of welfare state known as liberal democratic.[18] In contrast to the other types, liberal welfare states are founded on the principle of a fundamental separation between the domains of state and society, a boundary that puts the state in a secondary position to the demands and needs articulated by social actors, whether through organized groups or representative political institutions. Liberal welfare states are therefore less inclined to display centrally directed intervention than their social democratic counterparts (Ruggie 1984). Governments in liberal welfare states seek to intervene minimally in the market; intervention is undertaken in order to compensate for adverse consequences of market forces or private-sector activities, but not so much as to redirect the market or the private sector. State intervention is intended neither to supersede market forces nor to dictate or direct the conduct of private affairs, merely to enable them to return to a condition of "normalcy" (Gutmann 1988; Moon 1988). Liberal welfare states rarely succeed in adhering to these principles of intervention, however. Instead of merely correcting social problems and then stepping back, government intrusions tend to be deeper than intended and difficult to discontinue once instituted. The primacy of separate spheres requires that the state specify the reasons for its intervention. Since each specification evokes its own regulatory mechanism, the result is, paradoxically, ever more intrusive intervention (Ruggie 1992). Thus, although keeping the domains of state and society separate is fundamental to a liberal order, roles and relations oscillate between the society-centric and state-centric models.

Much of the literature on liberal welfare states contrasts their features with other forms of welfare states, particularly with social democratic systems, in which state intervention more positively directs the flow of market and private-sector forces and in which state regulatory activities are pronounced (Esping-Andersen 1990). Therefore, these discussions often emphasize society-centric configurations in liberal welfare states as opposed to the state-centric model prevalent in social democracies. When individual countries are studied more closely, summary characteristics of the typologies often yield to variations on categorical themes.[19] And within-group studies are bound to find considerable deviations from the standard type (for studies of liberal welfare states, see Myles 1989 and Orloff 1993). My study seeks to investigate nuances in newly emerging state/society relations. It is an endeavor that is best conducted within a similar type of welfare state, to reduce the effects of ideological and political factors, rather than across types, where analysis often focuses on ideological and political factors. In this study, important differences emerge among the three countries despite their similar roots. But we will also see that they remain liberal welfare states nevertheless.

If dismantling of the welfare state were to occur anywhere, it would be in the United States, and to a somewhat lesser extent in Britain and Canada, because the roots of these liberal welfare states have been weaker than those in the social democracies of Western Europe. However, all three survived retrenchment. In addition, although the constitutive division between state and society remains fundamental, government actors in these three countries have begun to experiment with novel forms of cooperation with other social actors. Attempts to cope with economic uncertainties are no doubt motivating a search for creative solutions to social problems. Although all three governments are doing less themselves, especially in terms of provision, they are nevertheless generating more societal activity in the provision of social services. This study elaborates these newly emerging roles and relations and contrasts them with the persistence of older types of behavior.

Health Care in Three Liberal Welfare States

The empirical focus of this study is health care policy. Despite their similarity as liberal welfare states, Britain, Canada, and the United States have very different health care systems, which is to be expected to some extent. However, as the chapters that follow demonstrate, different empirical policies and programs can conform to the similarities captured by broad typologies of welfare states—the core structural features that persist despite the immediacy of everyday events. Focusing on one policy area raises questions of generalizability, which at first glance might seem especially problematical for the case of health care. For example, the National Health Service (NHS) in Britain is sometimes considered as an outlier in the British welfare state, because state intervention is deeper in health care than in other social programs. Chapter 6 examines these three health care systems in relation to other social policies. It shows, for one, that the NHS is not as much of an outlier as popular perception would have it, mainly because the NHS receives no more funding proportionate to GDP (gross domestic product) than other social programs. In contrast, Medicare and Medicaid expenditures in the United States exceed those on other social policies save education. Nevertheless, one might ask how representative government efforts in the field of health care are for U.S. welfare state activities when a substantial part of that field is constituted by the private sector. My response is that what the state is doing in health care tells us more than a little about welfare state issues, and especially because the U.S. government is currently engaged in major changes that are affecting the entire system of health care. Chapter 7 also addresses the uniqueness of health care development in the welfare state. Finally, my focus on liberal welfare states and the generalizability of my study to changes in "the" welfare state may be challenged. Rather than making claims of generalizability, my study is oriented toward identifying a new phenomenon in state/society relations. Whether or not this phenomenon is particular to the cases presented here can only be determined by further research; accordingly, all claims offered in this study are qualified and all references to "the state" ought to be considered circumscribed.[20]

Because health care costs have risen inexorably in recent years in all the advanced industrial societies, many governments have taken drastic measures to try to reduce expenditures. Retrenchment in health care contains many of the ambiguities that characterize welfare states in general. For instance, as governments in Britain, Canada, and the United States attempt to reduce their burden of provision, they are having to make very difficult choices about who should receive health care and under what circumstances. As a result, both public awareness and public involvement are increasing in debates about what health care should consist of, for whom, and where the decision making ought to take place. In addition, as state actors perform intermediary functions and as they collaborate with other social actors, the role of the state is coming to be based, less than in the past, on reaction to social demands or intervention in societal domains. The state is performing new roles, and as it does so, it is inducing other social actors to reconsider the validity of former assumptions about the terms of health care and their own roles in providing health care.

To examine this transformation in state and societal roles and relations in the three health care systems under study, I compare the evolution of prevailing patterns of decision making in health care policy. In the past, governments in Britain, Canada, and the United States responded to the demands of physicians and public opinion with increased provision (be it for hospital construction or cancer research), thereby exemplifying some features of the society-centric model. All three governments also attempted various kinds of intervention aimed at containing expenditures, including controls on physician fees or limits on treatment sessions, thereby exemplifying some features of the state-centric model. Both of these forms of activity are continuing. But at the same time, we are witnessing changes in the usual patterns of response as governments, health care providers, and recipients confront unprecedented dilemmas in health care that require greater cooperation. For instance, physicians and government actors are collaborating on timing the dissemination of new knowledge about human genome mapping, hoping to protect patients from anxieties about untimely deaths before therapies or even cures for some disorders are available. Meanwhile, some patients shun the thought of being kept alive under any circumstances and ask assistance from both physicians and government actors in writing "living wills" to protect their definition of human dignity. Are these responses related to retrenchment? Are they simply adaptations to cost control imperatives? Are not different concepts needed to capture what is going on?

To better understand ongoing changes in health care and health care policy, we need to go beyond the abstract formulations of state/society roles and relations contained in the three models discussed earlier. We need to specify more clearly who does what, and how, in the provision of care. I propose to do this by introducing an analytical framework for the study of "policy regimes."

The term *regime* is most commonly used in the welfare state literature to distinguish different types of welfare states. For instance, Esping-Andersen (1990) discusses three "regime-type clusters" or three "worlds of welfare capitalism": liberal, corporatist, and social democratic. I am examining only one type of welfare state. My application of the term *regime* is closer, therefore, to the more generic definition used in the international relations literature. Krasner has defined regimes as "sets of implicit or explicit principles, norms, rules, and decision-making procedures around which actors' expectations converge" in a given issue area (1983:2). I define a policy regime as a set of principles and norms of state/society roles, relations, and modes of decision making—for the present study, in the issue area of health care policy. I distinguish three types of policy regimes, corresponding to the three models of state/society roles and relations discussed earlier. But I go further than these models in specifying instrumentalities for the responses of state and social actors to current changes in health care. The main actors in these regimes are government decision makers, medical providers, and consumers (patients and insurance companies). Which of these are the actual purchasers of health care varies across the countries and over time. Table 1.1 summarizes the ideal typical characteristics of the three policy regimes.

TABLE 1.1 *Policy Regimes in Liberal Welfare States*

	ROLES	RELATIONS	DECISION MAKING
Segmented	Traditional division of rights and responsibilities	State secondary to society Respect for separate domains	Market rationality Constitutional separation of powers
Interventionist	State issuance of regulations, legislation challenged	Contentious	Technical rationality Subject to contested interpretations
Integrative	State supervision, facilitation of broader base of social action	Coordinated Respect for alternative perceptions, values	Substantive rationality Negotiated, consensual

The term *segmented policy regime* refers to a situation in which roles, relations, and decision making are based on a traditional division of authority, exhibiting the fundamental bifurcation of state and society that is a classic characteristic of liberal welfare states. This policy regime depicts a condition in which governments hesitate to intervene in the affairs of private social actors because social relations are based on the norm of respect for the fundamental division of rights and responsibilities between state and social actors. In the field of health care policy, a segmented regime separates independent bases of power between central and local units of government, on the one hand, and government and the medical profession, on the other. Segmentation in health care relations describes a situation in which the role of government is essentially to fund some portion of provision and the role of decentralized and/or professional actors is to decide how funds are to be expended and to implement those decisions. The mode of decision making thus reflects the separate domains of authority and competence. This functional division of labor tends to be justified on legal/constitutional grounds.[21]

A segmented policy regime survives best in a context of economic growth in which no set of actors needs to challenge seriously the legitimate domain of another set of actors. Self-maximizing proclivities of any one set of actors do not generally impinge on others when sustained by a growing economy. In addition, a growing economy supports a broad understanding of the general purpose of health care provision, such as improvement in health outcome, which benefits all social actors. However, even in times of economic growth, governments and sometimes other social actors have worried about ever-increasing health care costs and expenditures. In all three countries under study new policy instrumentalities began to appear as economic growth slowed in the 1970s and constrained the maximization of health care.

An *interventionist policy regime* typically occurs in liberal welfare states when segmented modes of decision making and policy implementation fail to achieve desired goals. Economic decline exacerbates such failure. An interventionist policy regime may begin with the need for government to do something to correct market failures or stem economic decline. Eventually, in an interventionist policy regime government actors identify social malfeasants and assert governmental power over them, attempting to change their behavior through legislation or penalties. The result is the "paradox of liberal intervention": Governments engage in a greater depth of intervention than foreseen or intended, thereby raising criticisms of an overbearing welfare state and reassertions of private spheres of authority.

In all three countries under study the sheer force of state intervention has been tempered by appeals to technical rationality. To reduce contestations, state intervention is justified, for example, by complex data on out-of-control expenditures pointing to specific errants or by projections of the problems that would result were activities left unregulated. Social relations are more adversarial in an interventionist than in a segmented policy regime. Thus, governmental resort to technical rationality may be countered by other kinds of information or by sheer political or expert power on the part of decentralized and professional actors who are the subject of regulations. In this way, the exercise of state power may be contained or even reversed, placing central government on the defensive, with decentralized and/or professional actors controlling expenditure and other decisions that define the parameters of health care. An interventionist policy regime is unstable, because liberal welfare states are ultimately based on respect for the separation of state and societal power and authority. However, in its pure form an interventionist policy regime operates on the principle that roles are based on knowledge or other sources of competence (compared to the traditional or market-based assignments of a segmented regime); that social relations are structured by regulatory legislation, which justifies government intervention into the social order; and that decision making involves technical rationality more than free-market rationality.

One of the goals of my study is to identify and explore the parameters of a possible third policy regime, in which the role of the state in health care provision may appear at first glance to be less active than before, when measured as expenditure or delivery, but in which the state, in fact, has adopted a new role of inducing other social actors to become more involved in health care provision. Adapting Mishra's term, I call this type of policy regime *integrative*. In this policy regime the state assumes a leadership role. The goals toward which the state leads other actors are not of its own making; they are constructed together with other social actors. In all the policy regimes, state actors are attempting to influence the

actions of others. The main differences are that in a segmented policy regime state efforts consist of proddings and appeals, and in an
interventionist policy regime they rely more on power and coer-
cion. In both of these regimes those toward whom state efforts are
directed resist change. In an integrative policy regime the terms of
social change are negotiated and become more mutually supportive
than in the other two regimes. My use of the term *integrative* thus
differs from Mishra's.[22]

In addition, the main characteristics of an integrative policy
regime center on the use of what Weber referred to as *substantive
rationality* on the part of all relevant actors in defining the principles and norms underlying their respective roles, relations, and
decision-making arrangements. According to Weber, substantive
rationality involves "some criteria of ultimate values" (Roth and
Wittich, eds., 1978:85), that is, moral ethics as compared to market
or technical rationality.

To be sure, "ultimate values" exist in both segmented and
interventionist policy regimes. In particular, the traditionalism of
a segmented policy regime could be considered an ultimate value.
But within a segmented policy regime, resort to traditional values
tends to be prescriptive and formulaic. Moreover, within segmented policy regimes state and social actors often resolve problems on the basis of market rationality, which consistently grants
supremacy to individual freedom of choice over social norms and
to the market over the state. Similarly, the role of ultimate values
in interventionist policy regimes is frequently displaced by technical rationality. For example, the utility of saving a life may be
calculated according to a cost-benefit analysis of the patient's
future contribution to productivity. Neither segmented nor interventionist policy regimes contain the sort of flexibility in choosing among ultimate values that is necessary to answer the complex and pressing questions that have arisen in contemporary
health care.

As state and social actors confront current dilemmas, they are
increasingly turning to various "criteria of ultimate values," such
as the meaning of human dignity or the responsibilities of social
collectivities, as well as to various methods of sorting out these
values. Which values and methods pertain cannot be stated in the
abstract, for they vary across time or place and according to the situation. What a doctor, patient, and family decide is best in one case

is not necessarily best in another case. The role of the state in such decision making is to assure that all views are represented and that none dominates in advance. In all cases, the processes that guide decision making are organic and the outcome represents an integration of prior differences among the relevant actors. The state may implement its role through review panels, courts, or public debate. An integrative policy regime suggests an authoritative state, but the state's use of its authority depends on the relations among the actors involved—that is, the state's role is greater when decisions are more conflictual, less when actors are in agreement. A more open-ended set of norms informs my concept of an integrative policy regime as compared to segmented or interventionist regimes.

In an integrative policy regime the determination of who should perform what roles is based on a more even distribution of power among the main actors than occurs in the other policy regimes. Thus, a stronger and surer starting point for the division of labor occurs than under conditions of asymmetry. In addition, resources are more exchangeable and rights and responsibilities more flexible. The capacities of state and social actors are therefore utilized for the task at hand. Yet there is no predicting the outcome of decisions. No set of actors—governmental, medical, legal, religious, familial, or even individual—holds the power of predetermination. Integrative policy regimes encourage the construction of forums for airing alternative values and for mediating among them to resolve dilemmas.

My concept of an integrative policy regime also reveals the complexity of economic variables in the contemporary welfare state. As I argued earlier, retrenchment has had mixed results, in which selective expansion has been as likely as cutbacks. Actors are as likely to increase spending as to practice self-restraint. Within an integrative policy regime, alternative, nonmarket, and nontechnical criteria justify expenditure decisions. When actors appeal to the scarcity of resources or denounce economistic measurements, they inevitably do so in terms of broader goals and substantive justifications, whether based on collective well-being or on individual integrity. The attempt to harmonize competing claims in terms of more universalistic norms distinguishes an integrative policy regime from the asymmetry of roles and relations in both segmented and interventionist regimes.

Conclusion

An integrative policy regime is far from a reality in health care in the three welfare states under study, and I make no claims that it exists. But its characteristics are discernible and its possibility thereby suggested. If some form of integrative policy regime is indeed emerging—one in which state and social actors are engaging in greater degrees of accommodation, cooperation, and collaboration—what does this say about the authority of the state? As we shall see, within an integrative policy regime the state not only retains its constitutional authority, but also can become more authoritative as it fosters integration among social actors. This kind of authority is different from that in segmented and interventionist policy regimes. It has different sources of power and different manifestations. In the country chapters I elaborate on what constitutes state authority in the contemporary welfare states of Britain, Canada, and the United States. The factors vary empirically by country, as does the extent to which government actors in the three countries have seized the opportunities offered by changes in the field of health care, but the possibility of an integrative policy regime is present in all three.

I find that these policy regimes have appeared in a similar order in the three countries. However, the appearance of any one does not necessarily displace the others.[23] Indeed, in all three countries under study one can discern the coexistence of all three regimes—to the extent that the suggestion of an integrative regime is valid. That segmented policy regimes appeared first is understandable, insofar as this type of regime describes the classic features of liberal welfare states. It is also understandable that interventionist policy regimes followed, insofar as their appearance in the 1970s and 1980s coincided with a period of economic decline, during which government actors undertook concerted efforts to control expenditures and decisions about social provision. Understanding the emergence of integrative policy regimes is one main analytical focus of this study. Insofar as the parameters of an integrative policy regime clarify the current anomaly of the welfare state, I will specify how its possible contours differ from features of both segmented and interventionist regimes. As the country chapters show, the fact that integrative policy regimes are very recent may explain why their operation has frequently faltered, causing state and social actors to revert to older methods of problem solving.

All three countries are undertaking novel approaches to health care issues, and their experiments cannot be characterized according to standard liberal welfare state criteria. By imputing the emergence of a similar policy regime, based on the integrative model, to capture these novel approaches, I am not suggesting that specific responses to health care dilemmas in the three countries are identical. The policy regime framework is typological and theoretical; it identifies core features of roles and relations that can pertain to different empirical correlates of health care provision and delivery. But common to the health care systems within each policy regime are the underlying principles, norms, and modes of decision making characteristic of that policy regime. These tie Britain, Canada, and the United States together as three liberal welfare states, each attempting to perform its tasks under new constraints.

The next three chapters present the evolution from segmented to interventionist to, possibly, integrative policy regimes, in Britain, Canada, and the United States, respectively. Chapter 5 discusses what could be construed as a counterargument to my notion of an integrative policy regime, namely, the suggestion that privatization best captures current changes. Privatization is taking place, but not at the expense of integrative modalities. Chapter 6 summarizes empirically the main features of health care in the three countries. Chapter 7 explores two alternative explanations for these developments—that the changes presented in this study are unique to health care because its technologically induced dilemmas are more profound than occur in other fields of social policy and that the welfare state has reached the limits of its growth within a global economy.

NOTES

1. American conservatives relish citing the founding fathers' denouncement of "Big Government." Douglas even found an appropriate phrase from Woodrow Wilson: "A history of liberty is the history of the limitations of government powers, not the increase of it" (1989:7–8). Accordingly, one of his chapters is entitled "Freedom Works."

2. According to O'Connor (1973), government expenditure is necessary, on the one hand, for the accumulation function. Governments facilitate capital accumulation through public expenditure on the economic infrastructure (transport systems, utilities); on the costs of reproducing labor (education, social services); and on research and development projects that help maintain

the foundations for capitalist expansion. On the other hand, most of these same state expenditures, but especially those for education and social services, are also necessary for the legitimation function. Whatever the state does to win and maintain mass support is part of its legitimation function, which both masks the primacy of the accumulation function in a capitalist system and serves as a mechanism for controlling the potential outbreak of class conflict endemic in capitalist society.

3. Some neo-Marxists maintained that contradictory state activities do not necessarily create full-fledged crises (Offe 1984). These theorists suggested that each stalemate contains a partial and temporary resolution but that in each such resolution contradictions intensify.

4. Brown (1988:7) argues that there has been an "uncoupling of social and macroeconomic policy, a marked departure from the attempted coordination between these two policies that was so prominent in the expansion of the post-war welfare state." But this assessment of one of the founding idea systems behind the welfare state does not mean that the welfare state in general is on its deathbed. Brown continues his analysis to show that the greatest restraints in social welfare spending occurred in services, not transfers. The implication is that governments can more easily curtail service programs over which they have more control than transfer payments that are subject to consumer forces. Governments can devise reductions in transfer payments, but these are more likely to be indirect and their consequences less visible less quickly. Administrative flexibility derived from the institutional structure of individual welfare states can also, then, account for the continuation of unemployment and pension payments. And insofar as social provision continues, the welfare state persists.

5. Therborn (1987) posits a "logic of market economies" argument, stating that capitalist markets require state institutions and that state intervention is a "functional necessity" to protect market processes. The argument is reminiscent of Polanyi's (1944) pronouncement that laissez-faire was planned. Therborn contrasts bourgeois welfare states with a state-centric proletarian type.

6. For example, the growing numbers of elderly citizens are exerting an inexorable force on state spending and program development (Pampel and Williamson 1985). Using OECD data, Klein and Scrivens (1985) found that the demographic push accounts for about one-third of the growth rate in social spending. Since programs for the elderly were among the first to be established when welfare states developed, functionalists have also argued that the strength of institutionalization as well as the length of institutional experience accounts for the programs' survival (Wilensky 1975)—even during periods of retrenchment.

7. Some studies show that expenditure decisions are mediated by such political factors as left-leaning governments and supportive public opinion (Hicks and Misra 1993). Such studies advance the basic pluralist vision of the state as secondary to society, with government actors responding to the needs and demands presented by social actors.

8. The neopluralists in this group differ from their traditional counterparts in their ambivalence about assessing the welfare state as overstretched, pri-

marily because they do not want to see social expenditures further reduced. They seek a redistribution of spending away from state-run services toward mechanisms that enable nonstate sectors to expand their role in welfare provision. These neopluralists maintain that the regulatory role of the state ought to continue but that it should be less restrictive and more facilitative of the efforts of social actors. They argue that all relevant actors should be involved in social provision, be they employees of providers or friends and relatives of recipients. Neopluralists offer little insight into methods for resolving conflicting interests among the various participants, however, for they assume that the process of dispersing power creates new legitimate bases of power: "participation, as a means to such ends, becomes an end in itself" (Higgins 1978:125).

9. Exactly what the state should do remains vague: "the state would cease to be the main provider of welfare but would continue as the main source of finance, and its regulatory role would increase. Thus welfare pluralists see the state as having more than a residual role. However, the state they have in mind is a decentralized one" (Johnson 1987:176). We are left wondering, therefore, how regulation facilitates decentralization and why the state's continuing role in financing social projects no longer carries the power to direct social actors as it once did.

10. Corporatism reemerged in the 1970s as a social scientific construct to explain the prominence of so-called peak associations (labor and business) in state decision making. Neocorporatists have set as their task the development of a theory of state/society roles and relations that is distinct from corporatism's foundation in fascism, on the one hand, and its affinity with pluralism, on the other. Unlike the authoritarian role of the state in fascism, neocorporatists conceptualize an authoritative state that guides societal decision making. And unlike the competitive role of interest groups in pluralist systems, neocorporatists conceptualize highly organized groups engaging in interest intermediation or concertation. Although neocorporatists usually favor a more neo-Marxist view of the crisis, they also critique the more orthodox Marxist position that the state reflects class interests and acts ultimately to secure the interests of the dominant, capitalist class. The main focus of the neocorporatist position is the transformation of class in contemporary society and the displacement of class interests by corporate interests. To put the distinction in Cawson's (1982) terms, class groups are characterized by their hierarchical position in the economy, corporate groups by their function in the economy. There is insufficient analysis, however, of the link between corporate interests and class interests. Therefore, a confluence of interests among social groups is assumed rather than studied.

11. See also Cawson (1986). In thus claiming that corporatism arises out of liberal capitalism, Cawson aligns himself with neo-Marxist theorists who refute any independence of the state from the economy. In contrast, Pahl and Winkler (1974), for example, claim that corporatism does not develop within capitalism but is a distinct form of economic structure constituting an alternative or sequel to capitalism. Also, in emphasizing a "facilitative" role on the part of the state, Cawson depicts a weak form of corporatism compared with

Winkler (1976), for example, who analyzes a shift from a supportive to a "directive" role for the state in the economy.

12. As Cawson continues his analysis, he turns to demonstrating that the role of the state has become weaker in relation to corporate groups. The argument rests on his claim that once policies have been decided, corporate groups, not the state, become the agents of policy implementation. And in exercising their powerful roles, corporate groups exacerbate the problems of a dual state. Organizations outside of parliament engage in corporatist politics, while a perfunctory parliament sits merely to represent individual and group interests. This fragmentation of the state lays the foundation for economic crisis, insofar as spending is fuelled by the bargains struck by elites. Cawson links the goals of professionals with those of public employees who have developed their own interests in further expanding public expenditure. Together they form a powerful corporate group governing the field of social policy. And because of the supremacy of peak associations in corporate politics and the consequent erosion of parliamentary politics, their demands are structurally immune to competition from other interest groups.

Cawson decries the attrition of democracy under corporatism, in the process of policy-making and policy implementation as well as in society more generally. He holds that since corporatism embodies a rationality based on the calculation of interests, it can only be reined in by alternative forms of rationality, based on norms and values. We must await, Cawson claims, the return of democratic norms as the core of society's institutions, achieved through the practice of democracy at the individual level. His recommendation retreats, in the end, to the solipsism of classical liberalism, but the lament for a moral dimension in social politics is moving and reminiscent of the early British classics. For instance, Marshall (1950) emphasized the concept of social rights in the development of the welfare state. Titmuss (1968) argued that greater equality would only come about through concerted efforts by government actors to develop and implement purposeful social policies.

13. Such inconsistency muddies the systematic understanding and use of the concept of corporatism in the literature. For critiques see Martin (1983) and Williamson (1985).

14. The distinction is with a differentiated welfare state, which resulted from a postwar consensus about the role of the state, based on a fusion of the ideas of Keynes and Beveridge. The term *differentiation* is intended to convey the basic liberal disposition of a constitutive separation of economy and polity, and hence to portray social programs as bifurcated and inadequate. A differentiated welfare state does not interfere with the supply side of economic behavior; instead, it relies on the regulation of demand and allows market forces to direct developments. Nor does a differentiated welfare state interfere with the agreements reached by society's peak associations, particularly the income bargains struck by labor and business. Interest groups compete for power in the state arena, and the social provisions emerging from a differentiated welfare state reflect the outcome of this competition. Since different interests win at different times, the gamut of social measures existing at any one time is fragmented, both reflecting and maintaining the competitive basis of

social relations. Mishra (1984:105) claims that the differentiated welfare state is a "step forward from a largely laissez-faire economy and residual welfare"; how this is so is unclear. However, Mishra places corporatism within the context of liberal market society, as does Cawson.

15. On this point Mishra falls back on social Keynesianism and on an expansionist view of the welfare state. He postulates collective responsibility in such an integrated system, but it is similar to the classic Keynesian consensus: "employers recognize full employment as a social objective while workers accept the need for wage moderation and higher productivity as a prerequisite for economic growth and social welfare" (1984:104).

16. Although Cawson conceptualizes a weaker form of corporatism than Mishra, both clearly distinguish corporatism from pluralism and authoritarianism. For Cawson, corporate interests do not automatically mesh with the state's interests; the state must act to create the meshing. For Mishra, the consensual, cooperative basis of interest articulation converts the state into one among several actors, but the one most able to facilitate concertation. In clarifying these distinctions, however, both Cawson and Mishra steer the concept of corporatism closer to another of its nemeses: managerialism. Under the managerial politics that develop in a corporatist system, shared purposes are more efficiently achieved by means of controls and decrees than by the rule of law (O'Sullivan 1988:23). Because political accountability is subsidiary in managerial politics, constitutional or other democratic restraints on elites are minimal, whether these check the actions and goals of the state and its accomplices or the organizations whose interests rule.

17. These aggregations commonly include expenditures for pensions, health care, and unemployment, and occasionally, education and income maintenance programs, for the top eighteen advanced industrial societies (measured in terms of social expenditure as a percent of GDP). It is now assumed that all these eighteen countries are welfare states—there is no nil category among them. The variations among them are a major focus of scholarly interest.

18. Therborn (1987:186) classifies these countries as market-oriented.

19. Recall those studies of the American welfare state discussed earlier that added to our understanding of state-centric features within this liberal democratic exemplar.

20. See Ragin (1987), especially Chapter 3, for further discussion of the problems faced by qualitative, small-number, case-oriented comparative research, as well as a vindication of the usefulness of this type of research and a discussion of its unique strengths in examining constellations, configurations, and conjunctures.

21. These latter characteristics provide a regularity that distinguishes my formulation of a segmented regime from Mishra's depiction of a differentiated welfare state in which competition and inconsistent wins and losses prevail.

22. The main difference is that Mishra's integrated welfare state rests essentially on an integration of social and economic policy and is thus a variant of the Keynesian welfare state (see note 15). In my model, economic considerations do not necessarily determine choices. Decision making is based on substantive rationality, and the integration is among varieties of values.

23. An analogy might be made to Weber's three types of authority. Although only one type of authority prevails in a particular historical era, the others are not entirely absent. Much of the scholarly debate about Weber's typology focuses on the contemporary form of legal-rational authority and on whether it obliterates opportunities for traditional and charismatic types to reappear, however tainted they may be by modernity.

Chapter Two

Britain

Britain's National Health Service (NHS) is a classic example of a fully nationalized system of health care delivery and provision. Inaugurated in 1948, earlier than national programs in most other European countries, its successes and failures have informed the direction of policies adopted elsewhere. The prototypical characteristics of the NHS include government dominance in the administrative and fiscal dimensions of health policy-making and implementation, and universal access to comprehensive health care services for all residents of the United Kingdom, funded by compulsory contributions to general revenue. This first glance at the NHS grounds it within an interventionist policy regime. Although the assessment is valid, this chapter also demonstrates that for most of NHS history the central government has not exerted a dominating command over health care. In fact, the central government has struggled for decades with other main actors in British health care to gain control over the allocation of resources. Much trial and error has gone into the effort to enhance the capacity of the state to harness the centrifugal forces of the separate powers and interests that for decades structured a segmented policy regime. The

main body of this chapter presents the evolution from a segmented policy regime, in which health care was organized by the distinct roles of government and other societal (mostly medical)
actors and by the tradition-bound relations between them, to an
interventionist policy regime, in which state actors attempted to
exert control over the factors of health care provision. The installment of an interventionist policy regime did not, however, eliminate features of segmentation, for Britain remains to this day a liberal welfare state.

At the same time, we can see in Britain the first signs of an integrated policy regime, signaling the survival of the British welfare
state after an era of retrenchment under conservative governments.
We have become accustomed to hearing of Britain's economic
woes, expecting a dismantling of its welfare state, and inferring a
retreat from original goals. My case for the emergence of an integrative policy regime focuses on the collaborative roles and relations that have developed in recent years between state and social
actors in British health care. I argue that although the state in
Britain has come to do less itself in terms of actual provision and
although what was done previously by the central government
alone is now in the hands of decentralized and nonstate actors, the
state is performing the essential role of overseeing a broader base
of provision.

In this new role the central government is exercising considerable authority over health care provision, even though it no longer
decides on the substance of provision. Past struggles with decentralized government units, known as local health authorities, and
with providers, both hospitals and doctors,[1] over the allocation of
limited NHS resources have given way to new modes of decision
making. Expenditure decisions remain a core issue surrounding the
distribution of power and authority in health care; however, the
rules governing these decisions are now formulated more collectively. The thesis of this book—that the welfare state is continuing
to evolve with a more authoritative though less visibly active state
at its core—is thus portrayed in the case of Britain as the achievement of decades of experimentation in responding to the exigencies
of defining authority over the political, economic, and social dimensions of health care.

I distinguish three broad phases in the evolution of policy regimes in British health care. Each phase exhibits an attempt on the
part of central government to develop an alternative strategy of

controlling resource allocation in the NHS. In the first phase, from 1948 to approximately 1962, the central government acted primarily as funder and facilitator of the system as a whole and succeeded in establishing central control over the outer limits of the NHS budget. However, ultimate authority for spending and for key decisions in resource allocation rested with the medical profession and to a less consequential extent with local authorities. Roles, relations, and decision making were thus segmented, with a deep-seated recognition of separate spheres of power and authority. Thus, although the creation of the NHS was an act of supreme intervention, the roles and relations that followed conformed to traditional patterns.

The second phase spans three decades of a rise, crest, and transformation in an interventionist policy regime. In the 1960s government actors adopted the tools of macroplanning in an effort to exercise greater direction over resource allocation. Although planning as such did not fully take root, it established an expanded bureaucracy to handle the increased flow of information presupposed by a planning rationale. Relations between state and social actors became more adversarial with the introduction of intervention through microplanning and management in the 1970s. Government actors became more proficient in applying administrative techniques to improve efficiency and effectiveness. They tried to co-opt the medical profession into the decision-making apparatus of the NHS, but the results proved fruitless and the medical profession retained final determination of the philosophy of the NHS. The medical profession's power over expenditure decisions began to recede, however, in the 1980s, when the central government adopted stronger measures of control over resource allocation. Earlier techniques of management became more sophisticated, and an ethos of efficiency came to prevail to the point of dominating the philosophy of the NHS. The conservative rhetoric of the era masked an underlying transformation that was astir in the roles and relations between providers and payers. The temper of the times facilitated an unprecedented assertion of authority by the state.[2] Beginning in the early 1990s the NHS underwent the most fundamental transformation in its history. Although the changes appear to fulfill political goals of decentralization (and privatization), they actually mark the emergence of a more integrative system of roles, relations, and decision making.

Establishing a Modus Vivendi:
Separate Spheres of Control (1948–1962)

Creating the NHS was an act of compromise. Out of the ravages of World War II, a consensus emerged between state and social actors to implement the Beveridge Report proposals for a Keynesian welfare state in Britain, with health care as its "temple."[3] Behind this veneer of consensus, however, hard bargains had to be struck to reshape decades of practice without overstepping established boundaries of authority.

The main task in constructing the NHS was defining the precise roles of the central government, on the one hand, and of the local health authorities and the medical profession, on the other. This task involved a debate over not only nationalization per se, but also whether nationalized health care should be based on insurance or service. The 1911 National Health Insurance Act had established a national insurance system to pay general practitioners (GPs) to provide basic health care for a portion of the working population. Alongside this insurance system, local governments over the decades had painstakingly constructed a service model to provide public health care (e.g., immunization) to the population. The two systems, insurance and service, were not systematically linked. When Parliament was debating the organization of the NHS in 1944 and in 1946, it was confronted with a choice between an insurance system, favored by GPs,[4] and the service-based model, favored by local governments. In the end both sides won in principle. The NHS "reorganized but did not radically transform medical care in Britain" (Fox 1986:132). The compromise resulted in a cumbersome system. I briefly outline the cast of characters, their respective roles, and the relations between them before elaborating repeated efforts on the part of state actors to bring order to health care provision in the early years of the NHS.

Segmented Government

The most sweeping change brought about by the NHS in 1948 was the nationalization of all hospitals; only a few remained within the private sector (mainly for the upper class in London). Nationalization removed a large measure of control over hospital-based health care from local authorities and created instead new regional boards of governance whose members were appointed by the central government. Local health authorities were left with the still substantial responsibility for public health services and non-hospital health services (child welfare, district nursing, health centers, or clinics). Throughout the history of the NHS the balance of power between local health authorities and the centralized units of government (especially the Ministry of Health itself) has remained an area of controversy and debate. These relationships (and not those between the government and the medical profession) have also been the main object of the several restructurings in the NHS.

The main issue of contention in center/local relations—who would have control over what—was solved in the early days of the NHS by a functional division of labor. The central government was to maintain control of the overall system of health care, funding it through general taxation, and setting priorities and guidelines. One of the first and lasting achievements in establishing central control over the budget was the decision to cap NHS expenditures.[5] For their part, local health authorities were responsible for deciding which kinds and levels of services were to be provided. These demarcations evoke the principle of separate domains characteristic of a segmented policy regime. However, the separation was weak with regard to the relations between central and decentralized government actors. Central government in Britain, immersed in the civil service tradition, finds it difficult not to meddle in the microdecisions of local authorities to ensure that national priorities are being followed.[6] Thus, a typically British mode of governance appeared in these first years of the NHS: Circulars were sent from central government to inform local levels of new policies and remind them of existing ones. These circulars were generally advisory, offered details and examples of how to implement policies, but sometimes they mandated action and broached the possibility of greater central government intervention. In stopping short of active intervention, however, central government actors conceded that they could do no more than plead for policy implementation, thereby conforming to the norms of a segmented policy regime. By the mid-1950s, a form of "policy-making through exhortation" based on a plethora of circulars came to characterize intergovernmental relations in the NHS, and it reinforced segmentation (Klein 1983:51).

Within the central government itself, a decline in the status of the Ministry of Health shortly after the creation of the NHS not only weakened the center's ability to do anything more than exhort, but also left central government in a secondary, even passive relation to the demands and complaints coming from "the periphery" (Klein 1983:50–51). Local health authorities could more easily ignore central requests for information and demands for stricter vigilance when the center's power to follow up was lacking. Given the initial weakness of the central government, national uniformity in health care standards and provision was abandoned prematurely as a goal for the NHS, in favor of localism and consequent diversity in health provision. The result was a complicated and unwieldy "system" of health care provision. Despite their relative independence, local governments complained about too much central interference and about drowning in a stream of circulars. They thereby introduced an adversarial tone that strained intergovernmental relations for years. It did not erupt, however, until the next phase, when the central government no longer hesitated to intervene. Bevan was fond of saying that the NHS was framed for a "maximum of decentralization to local bodies [and] a minimum of itemized central approval" (Klein 1983:49–50). His words reflected sensitivity to traditional domains. But at the same time, they indicated awareness of the difficulties in maintaining separate spheres. Although significant in their own right, the problems in intergovernmental relations deflected attention from a more consequential thorn embedded in the NHS, namely, the inviolable authority of the medical profession.

Segmentation Between Profession and Government

From the preprofessional days of medical practice in Britain doctors were divided along class lines that defined not only their social and educational backgrounds but also their patients. The well-educated, elite physicians served the upper classes and were members of the prestigious Royal College of Physicians or Royal College of Surgeons. In contrast, the more lowly GPs provided basic apothecary and surgery (formerly barber) services. In 1832 a group of GPs based outside London protested the exclusiveness of the Royal Colleges by establishing the British Medical Association (BMA), a trade union type of organization that affirmed its members' worker status (Forsyth 1966:4–5). This basic division between GPs and elite physicians deepened with the growth of hospitals in the late nineteenth century. Only the more elite and increasingly more specialized physicians were associated with hospitals. Class criteria eventually gave way to area of knowledge as the basis of differentiation among doctors. The bifurcation between GPs and specialists has been troublesome for the state, complicating its efforts to control the medical profession as a whole and ultimately the NHS.

The 1911 National Health Insurance Act extended GP services to lower-paid workers who, along with their employers, contributed on a compulsory basis to a nationalized insurance fund.[7] The state paid GPs an annual fee for each person on their list (a system known as capitation). The 1911 Act also reinforced the evolving demarcation in the domains of GPs and hospital specialists: GPs treated patients in offices and community clinics, leaving hospitals for specialists. Besides the capitation fees, GPs received direct payment for services from noninsured persons. By 1940 about half of the working population, mainly manual workers but not their dependents, was covered by national insurance. Some of those not covered had private insurance. Those without any insurance used public hospitals, which refused care to no one.

During the wartime debate over the NHS, the BMA struggled to maintain the insurance basis of payment for GPs, who feared the loss of autonomy that might accompany salaried status. In the end, the minister of health, Aneurin Bevan, more committed to providing health services than to a particular method of paying doctors, conceded a separate place in the NHS for GPs, allowing them to continue to work much as before (Fox 1986:134.). The organization and jurisdictional boundaries of the local administrative units that registered and paid GPs changed somewhat, but the livelihood of GPs was unaffected.[8] In fact, under the NHS GPs fared significantly better on the whole: Their capitation fees were raised, doubling their average income from a decade earlier; their incomes were adjusted to inflation; and they no longer needed to employ collection agencies to hunt down fees owed by poor patients.

Specialists and consultants enjoyed a higher status than GPs from their early affiliation with the more prestigious Royal Colleges and later their association with hospitals.[9] Their activities in general were cast more broadly than those of GPs and included teaching and, for some, politics. Among themselves, specialists and consultants were stratified, with "surgeon princes," Harley Street specialists, and consultants in the famous teaching hospitals at the top of the hierarchy. But by the 1940s most specialists were finding their livelihoods strained by the growing expense of technologies for health care and the resulting dire financial conditions of hospitals, most of which were dilapidated at the conclusion of the war. Moreover, the fact that many hospital consultants were dependent on GPs for referrals was a further impediment to their security of employment. For these reasons, consultants were more receptive to the White Paper proposals for an NHS than were GPs.

With the nationalization of all hospitals under the NHS, consultants were brought under a nationalized system of salaried remuneration. It is important to note that, although their incomes came from the government, hospital consultants were "not regarded as servants of the State" (Forsyth 1966:28–29). They were specialists in their own right and under independent contract with the newly created regional hospital boards. They could choose to work full or part-time for the NHS while retaining private practices for private-paying patients. Most consultants chose the latter option, with varying amounts of time under NHS contract; only a few physicians chose to opt out of the NHS entirely. One important concession to consultants was allowing them to use private, so-called pay beds in public hospitals for their fee-paying patients. A system of "awards" was established to supplement any reductions in incomes for physicians who were fully or mostly affiliated with the NHS (Forsyth 1966:30).[10] These flexibilities in remuneration, together with the fact that the nationalization of hospitals guaranteed funding for medical care, improved the livelihood of most consultants without reducing the opportunities of any. Nor did nationalization itself pose any problems for consultants—they had already had a favorable experience with the national management of hospitals during the war, finding that "their control over administrative decisions" had increased (Fox 1986:133). The special status granted to teaching hospitals and, perhaps above all, the promise of clinical autonomy for all physicians, clinched their support for the NHS.

In the early days of the NHS, a clear deference to the authority of medical opinion on matters of health care permeated all aspects of

NHS organization. A statement made in Parliament by the postwar minister of health, Aneurin Bevan, assured doctors that they would command judgments on resource allocation: "the function of the Ministry of Health is to provide the medical profession with the best and most modern apparatus of medicine, and to enable them freely to use it, in accordance with their training for the benefit of the people of this country. Every doctor must be free to use that apparatus without interference from secular organisations" (Hansard 1946, col. 52). This deference and the clinical freedom that followed applied to both GPs and consultants. But its implications were more significant for the impact that hospital consultants would have on NHS funds. In the early years of the NHS, doctors did not need to include financial considerations in their medical decision making. It was the governing boards of hospitals that had to worry about the costs of medical decisions and present their accounts to government representatives. The power of the medical profession extended beyond the domain of clinical autonomy to include a measure of political power in deciding how to spend public monies. There was strong medical representation on the various boards of governance within the NHS. As Bevan also said in the speech just quoted: "I believe it is a wise thing to give the doctors full participation in the administration of their own profession" (Hansard 1946, col. 52).

In sum, a functional division of labor existed in the separate spheres of responsibility between GPs and consultants. Because of status differences, the mutuality of professional respect was asymmetrical. Moreover, salaried compensation had mitigated the reliance of hospital consultants on GPs for referrals. The everyday life of the NHS was more affected, however, by the separation between governmental and professional spheres. The functional division of labor whereby the government funded what the medical profession decided should be funded also involved an asymmetrical deference. It became increasingly more problematical as government's concerns about cost control evaded medical decision making. In contrast, professional demands for increased funding influenced governmental decisions, to the detriment of the economic health of the NHS. Government actors gradually learned to use their power of the purse, but this assertion of power became meaningful only when the economy began to falter.

Rising Costs, Falling Expectations

Before the NHS had been in operation for a full year, it became clear that Beveridge's original expectation—that demand for health services would taper off as needs were met—was in error. The first Ministry of Health report on the NHS indicated that every area of cost, from eyeglasses to salaries, exceeded original calculations. A debate ensued—indeed, one that continues to this day—as to why expenditures grew and whether they were justifiable. Blame was spread all around—on doctors, consumers, and the Ministry of Health. In the early years of the NHS, the ministry was convinced that rising expenditures were necessary to meet health care needs, and it encouraged spending, which, in turn, inflated the expectations of both the public and the medical profession (Fox 1986:141ff.).

The burden of undertaking solutions to the problem of rapidly increasing expenditures was widely distributed, but it did not include doctors. Instead, complaints by government actors that physicians had too much freedom to spend and too little incentive to economize were countered by medical assertions that the NHS needed more funds. Some politicians concurred with doctors and voiced the opinion that growing NHS expenditures were politically expedient. "Tinkering" adjustments in patterns of spending resulted, but they did little to restrict the prerogatives of clinical autonomy in expenditure decisions.[11] From its beginning, then, the NHS has represented a "bargain between the State and the medical profession. Although central government controlled the budget, doctors controlled what happened with that budget" (Klein 1983:82). As long as this modus vivendi prevailed, a segmented policy regime continued to structure the roles and relations of government and medical actors. Rising expectations about health care together with a sluggish economy rendered this policy regime unstable. However, insofar as governmental attempts to control the internal finances of the NHS evaded the domain of clinical autonomy, a segmented policy regime dragged on for decades.

Intervention Through Planning (1962–1982)

The central government has always claimed authority in principle over the global budget of the NHS. However, practical power over implementation has resided with both decentralized governmental actors and, more important, the medical profession. In the 1960s the central government began to develop and utilize new tools of governance. It was an era of planning in general in Britain.[12] In this phase, first macro- and then microplanning became the main tools that central government used to assert its power. As central government actors acquired experience, they were able to develop increasingly more sophisticated measures that constructed the principles and norms of an interventionist policy regime.

Central Intervention in Local Domains

Macroplanning

From the inception of the NHS local health authorities were responsible for the provision of public health and community services. In 1963 the Ministry of Health presented a set of ten-year plans for the development of community care in health and welfare services entitled *Health and Welfare: The Development of Community Care*. It was the first time that local authorities had engaged in any exercise in planning, so their projections of future needs tended to be "guesstimates" more than calculated plans (Allsop 1984:57). Nevertheless, the information demonstrated significant disparities in access and provision.

The desire to enlist local authorities in planning was rooted in the central government's goal of developing more uniform standards of health care across the nation. But the goal was poorly served by the means at hand. The macroplanning ventures initiated in the 1960s did not capture the sort of information required to assess the health care needs of the population, let alone to direct this information to improving provision. Moreover, the whole endeavor revealed that local authorities had considerable autonomy in making their own decisions about health care and that they, accordingly, resisted the loss of autonomy implicit in "planning." As a result, a revised Health and Welfare Plan presented in 1966 did no more than reiterate the continuing disparity in services across local authorities. Further plans and provisions for local authority health services faltered.

These first tentative steps by central government to intervene in the affairs of local governments brought to the fore deep-rooted problems in intergovernmental relations. To put it in terms of the policy regimes framework, the principle of separate domains that had informed roles and relations in an earlier era was no longer applicable in an era when central government actors sought to gain greater fiscal control over the NHS. By the late 1960s problems in intergovernmental relations in health and related social services led to a formal inquiry. A major commission, set up to "rationalize" local authority services, published the Seebohm Report in 1972.

A Planned Reorganization

The 1974 reorganization of the NHS, as outlined in the Seebohm Report, culminated past efforts to impose administrative logic on the NHS by unifying its three tiers (central, regional, and local) of administrative authority and introducing a more manageable top-down line of authority.[13] On paper at least, central control seemed possible. At the top of the hierarchy stood the Department of Health and Social Services (DHSS).[14] It issued its directives to fourteen new regional health authorities (RHAs).[15] Immediately below the RHAs were ninety newly created area health authorities (AHAs).[16] Finally, areas were divided into district health authorities (DHAs).[17] This reorganization reflected one of the central government's goals: that the new planning process combine greater local input (a bottom-up flow of information) together with observance of the new guidelines for national priorities (a top-down flow).

The prevailing view as well as the intent of the reorganized system was well captured by the slogan "maximum delegation downwards, matched by accountability upwards." It found expression both in the planning methodology and in the implementation of team management. These strategies for central government control indicated that national goals were to be achieved through central direction of decentralized activities, indicating that an interventionist policy regime had taken hold. Reorganization also allowed certain substantive goals to be articulated—above all, a redistribution of resources from the richer to the poorer parts of the country and from the better-funded to the struggling health services. How these goals were executed signals a transition from macro- to micromanagement.

Microplanning

Because earlier attempts at planning had done little to change entrenched inequities in access to and provision of health care, the Labour secretary of state for health and social services, Richard Crossman, set up a working party to consider specific mechanisms for improving the formulation and implementation of plans for equality in health care. The working party's report was presented in 1976; its recommendations remained the basis of resource allocation until they were formally dissolved in 1991. Known as the RAWP (Resource Allocation Working Party) formula, this set of measures offered a sophisticated methodology for calculating relative need and applying these calculations to resource reallocation. It represented a refinement in the technical tools of administration available to central government and enabled the central government to engage in an unprecedented form of micromanagement.[18]

The initial consequences of applying the RAWP formula revealed an underlying incompatibility between micro- and macromanagement. RAWP operated retrospectively, whereas the planning it was intended to facilitate was prospective (Paton 1985:30). Contradictions of this sort reflect a more general hesitancy on the part of liberal welfare states to intervene, which results, among other things, in stop-go patterns of intervention. Because liberal welfare states are uncomfortable with micromanagement, when it does occur it is inevitably flawed. Macromanagement fails as a result, because it is insufficiently complemented by micromanagement tools. RAWP was a technical input methodology unsupported by any mechanism of control. Adding to the problem, the RAWP methodology could not deliver the reductions in equalities it was designed to achieve.[19] Yet, despite these shortcomings, RAWP did achieve a measure of resource reallocation, and accordingly, government actors considered it a "perfectly acceptable attempt to assess differences in need and to compensate for them" (Allsop 1984:97–98). However, the reallocation was insufficient to improve health care and achieve better indicators of health outcomes. Behind the failure of the RAWP formula was a reluctance on the part of local governments to follow through on central government goals and provide adequate resources to health care provision. In part, local governments may have been reacting to a newfound resolve on the part of central government actors to implement a policy of redistribution without major expenditure increases. For their part central government actors were putting their recently acquired expertise to good use in enforcing a long-dormant goal for the NHS.

Reallocation Among Services

One specific area where microinterventionist planning was implemented was in the so-called Cinderella services. After a number of studies had revealed that services for the elderly, mentally handicapped, and mentally ill were severely underfunded relative to need and compared to acute hospital services, the central government adopted among its priorities a redistribution of funds to these services. Since they were all the responsibility of local levels of government, relations between local health authorities and local personal social service departments became a major issue in the goal of improving community care.

Central government actors attempted to redirect local government provision of community services by suggesting that local authorities conduct joint planning efforts with AHAs. To facilitate such efforts the DHSS set up joint staff consultative committees (later joint consultative committees) that were given special grants with which to implement joint services and projects.[20] The tasks of the committees and the intentions of central government were clearly laid out in several planning guides issued by DHSS and intended as consultative documents, not prescriptions.[21] However, the guides exhibited the difficulty of separating advice from prescription, especially on the part of a central government searching for more control. Central government actors envisioned planning as a two-way process. First, a central planning unit in DHSS set out the guidelines, established through Public Expenditure Survey Committee negotiations and the system of program budgeting, within which joint committees were to plan. Then the decentralized levels would fill in the details, which were sent back up the line to the DHSS. Finally, to keep track of and encourage health authority compliance with its priorities, the DHSS began to use program budgeting to allocate resources differentially among the health authorities. The central government had sharpened its tool of administration. And it added authority to its power by directing the tools toward a valued goal—improving equality in health care. The combination justified a significant measure of central intervention in the decision making of local governments.

But central government actors did not take full advantage of this opportunity to effect changes in health care provision. In the face of local authority resistance, they reverted to reacting to reassertions of traditional rights and responsibilities. Local governments had complained bitterly about the invasion of micromanagement and the very real costs it entailed if community services were to be improved. Also, as the local authority responses came back to DHSS, it became clear that wide variations among local units precluded adherence to specific targets for improving services. Accordingly, the DHSS relaxed its goals for national standardization, as reflected in a 1977 document entitled *The Way Forward*. According to Ham (1982:70–71), within a period of one year, it became apparent that the hoped-for national standards would be modified by the local authorities and the medical profession that advised them. Further planning guides reflected backtracking on specifying what was to be achieved and how. Instead, planning once again took the form of exhortation through DHSS circulars.

The Labour minister of health, Richard Crossman, who oversaw the preparatory stages of reorganization, had worried about the overcentralization and overbureaucratization implicit in the hierarchical structure of the newly reorganized NHS. But even he had wanted "effective central control over the money spent on the service . . . to ensure that the maximum value is obtained from it" (Haywood and Alaszewsky 1980:36). His Conservative successor, Sir Keith Joseph, was more open about his desire for "managerial efficiency" (central control over decentralized units) and clearer lines of accountability (from the decentralized units to the center). Some controls on overcentralization were useful, of course, to prevent too much responsibility (and therefore blame) being put on central government and to mitigate excessive delays in actions taken. Overcentralization, in the sense of overbearing central power, did not occur during this phase. Indeed, the 1974 reorganization and its goals of greater central control through first top-down and then bottom-up planning were widely seen as a "failure" (Klein 1983:15). For insights into future directions it is instructive to examine the reasons for this apparent failure.

There is a subtle contradiction among the various methods of intervention employed during this phase to achieve central control. The hierarchical structure of the NHS specified a clear chain of command on paper, but the planning process developed for the NHS was not an effective mechanism for implementing central control.

In and of itself, planning is more of an integrative and comprehensive undertaking than is expressed in a hierarchical command structure (Klein 1983:62). Moreover, the joint consultative committee format for developing planning gave considerable scope to local authorities to decide their own needs and areas of collaboration. And central government actors could not respond to local demands without compromising the central government's goal of cost containment. The goal itself had been only implicitly articulated, overtaken to some extent by the details of microlevel planning. And local desires (indeed needs) for more funding were all too clear. Central government initially interpreted local government difficulties in implementing planning as recalcitrance; accordingly, it reverted to tried-and-true methods of central governance. Therefore, out of frustration and because of traditional constraints, the penchant of the British government to issue directives through circulars resurfaced. This became a phase in which the promise of strategic management deteriorated into prescriptive management. Klein (1983) emphasizes the development of negotiation during this period; my sense is that what took place was more of a learning process about the role of sanctions and incentives in bargaining. It did not come to fruition until the next phase.

Government Intervention in Professional Domains

Macroplanning

Reflecting the new spirit of planning at Whitehall, a hospital plan presented in 1962 proposed revamping hospital care through centrally determined criteria of efficiency and rationality.[22] The plan set as its central goal construction of ninety new, large district general hospitals that would offer a full array of hospital services in a single setting to a substantial catchment population.[23] Although the plan also proposed upgrading some of the country's existing hospitals, it was expected that the district general hospitals would eliminate the need for smaller, less efficient local hospitals. The Hospital Plan melded the particular interests of the actors involved. From the government's standpoint, large hospitals could improve efficiency by concentrating resources and attaining economies of scale. Moreover, the government held a more specific measure of control over the allocation of resources by, for example, specifying the permissible number of beds per population. On the other side of the picture, however, potential government control was contradicted by the interests of the medical profession. Large hospitals granted doctors greater access to advanced technology, a costly prospect for government.

In the research study groups and conferences that preceded and informed the development of the Hospital Plan, not only opposing interests but alternative types of expertise were pitted against each other. Government representatives offered their measures of efficiency and effectiveness in hospital resource allocation. Representatives of the medical profession presented their vision of future health care with advanced hospital equipment. Perhaps because government actors were too inexperienced in the new methods of technical analysis or because their deference to doctors was deep, doctors won. Although the hospital plan represented a "marriage between professional aspirations and the new faith in planning" (Klein 1983:74), it was clear who had the upper hand. The "detailed recommendations of the Plan—the basic vision of what a hospital service should be like—were almost entirely determined by the medical [profession and] designed to maximize the quality of care" (Klein 1983:74). The terms of the marriage contract granted government the legal power to control expenditures. This power was not enough, however, to achieve the government's goals for the Hospital Plan. Planning and global budgeting were still too weak to budge the autonomy of providers—particularly the medical profession, which continued to define the modalities of health care. The government made one more attempt to influence medical decision making through planning.[24] Its failure revealed that government actors remained more comfortable with the status quo method of bringing doctors around to the philosophy of cost control through persuasion, education, and exhortation.

A change in emphasis began in the 1970s. In 1967 the Joint Working Party on the Organization of Medical Work in Hospitals was set up to enable clinicians "to appreciate fully the importance of their role in management problems" (Allsop 1984:60). Its report, known as the First Cogwheel Report, suggested a number of administrative changes in hospital services "in order to promote improved efficiency in the organization of medical work" (Haywood and Alaszewsky 1980:111).[25] It was hoped that increasing the involvement of doctors in decisions about hospital resource allocations would not only educate them but also improve coordination in activities and spending patterns within a hospital through collective control. It was expected that improved hospital planning would follow.

An assessment of the implementation of the First Cogwheel Report began within a few years and was presented in 1972 under the title *Management Arrangements in the Reorganized National Health Service* (the Grey Book). This Second Cogwheel Report noted with disappointment that fewer than half of the country's large hospitals had established Medical Executive Committees for joint decision making on resource allocation. Some hospitals had merely added the new committees to existing ones without any revamping. Rather than the hoped-for co-optation, doctors continued to consider the new committees as advisory only. Without any further incentives to do so, doctors were reluctant to assume managerial roles that might circumscribe the sanctity of individual clinical autonomy. The Second Cogwheel Report suggested that the problem of doctors' seeming lack of awareness of the cost implications of their decisions was "to be found as much in the attitude of mind of those who embrace change as in the structure they adopt" (Haywood and Alaszewsky 1980:114). So instead of assuming that individual members of the medical executive committees were responsible clinicians who make clinical decisions to the best of their judgment, the report emphasized the collegiate nature of medical practitioners and the collective basis of their knowledge.[26] The Second Cogwheel Report therefore called for increased consultation among all clinicians (including doctors and nurses) and for increased interdisciplinary coordination across divisions in hospitals. As Haywood and Alaszewsky (1980:115) put it:

> The objectives of [these] proposals for multi-disciplinary management teams were to formalize . . . co-option and thereby make the medical profession accept the burdens of and responsibility for power. The working party's hope was that the medical member on the management team would act as a representative of his colleagues who, having been involved in the process, would feel bound by the decisions.

The importance of the Cogwheel Reports lies in their preparatory groundwork for changing the roles of medical professionals and the consequent relations of medical and nonmedical actors in health care. More immediately, the reports paved the way for the introduction of management teams in the next phase. They set out in detail a new description of functions and structure for NHS administrative units that informed the upcoming reorganization of the NHS.[27]

Microplanning

The 1974 reorganization of the NHS contained an opportunity for the medical profession to maintain its authority over NHS expenditures. The reorganization implemented the recommendations of the 1972 Grey Book on *Management Arrangements in the Reorganized NHS* by setting up management teams consisting of administrators, medical professionals, and lay or consumer representatives. These management teams were established at regional, area, and district levels.[28] They were an attempt on the part of central government to use a form of co-optation to regulate local decision making and implementation of policies. But because of the design of the teams, it was the central government that came to be co-opted once again by the dominance of the medical profession. Although doctors did not initially approve of management teams, they were able to dominate decision making. The majority of members on the teams were from professional medical backgrounds, and the positions of chair and vice-chair were commonly shared by the two hospital consultants on the teams, deflating the presumption of multidisciplinary and consensual teamwork.[29] Nevertheless, although the implicit purpose of changing the structure of decision making away from medical dominance toward multidisciplinary criteria may have failed, the more deep-seated purpose of involving the medical profession in management issues took root. Government actors continued to assume that involvement in management would educate doctors not only about the cost implications of their medical decisions, but also about the style of governance entailed by management.

Besides these indirect efforts to involve doctors in NHS matters, the DHSS engaged in more direct intervention. In an attempt to influence the clinical practices of doctors, one of the 1976 planning guides contained a bibliography of reports on "innovations in clinical practices, including methods of treating patients on an outpatient basis rather than as inpatients, and ways of reducing the number of unnecessary X-rays carried out" (Ham 1982:155). The document stated that it sought to "encourage further scrutiny by the profession of the resources used by different treatment regimes" (DHSS 1976:28). This was the first time that a government report officially implicated medical decisions in the allocation of resources. No further attempts to influence doctors were made until the 1980s.

More pointed efforts by central government actors to exercise control over doctors occurred in two other issue areas: pay beds and contracts. The initial consensus creating the NHS had been forged around these issues; their reintroduction on the political agenda at this stage signaled the beginning of changing power relations. One major concession by the central government at the creation of the NHS was allowing doctors to admit their private-paying patients to specially set-aside beds in public hospitals. The Labour Party had constantly voiced opposition to pay beds, charging that doctors were exacerbating social inequalities by advancing their private-paying patients in treatment queues. Not until the 1970s, however, did Labour politicians act on their opposition, strengthened by the tools of intervention that government actors had developed and emboldened by the scandals on inappropriate use of pay beds publicized in the mass media. By the mid-1970s a Labour government began to introduce proposals to gradually reduce and eventually eliminate pay beds. It was replaced by a Conservative government before the phasing-out process could be completed, but doctors had felt the sting from this attempt to limit their prerogatives.

Central government has periodically sought to influence doctors by manipulating incomes, but rarely has intervention disturbed the tradition-bound separation of state/medical domains. For example, from the beginnings of the NHS, hospital consultants have been allowed to choose the extent of their association with the NHS. In the early days most had part-time contracts, in which more than half of their time was within the NHS and the remainder was reserved for private practice. By the 1970s, less than half of consultants worked at least part-time for the NHS. Differences among specialties indicated that lucrative opportunities for private practice and the amount of time doctors worked for the NHS were negatively correlated. To attract doctors back to the NHS, the Labour government introduced a system of merit awards for consultants who worked full-time for the NHS. The next Conservative administration appreciated the power of incentives in the merit award system less than the opportunity it provided to negotiate with consultants. It agreed to a new contract with consultants permitting private practice without loss of NHS earnings. In return, consultants agreed to self-police their queue-jumping practices (Klein 1983:135). Merit awards were maintained for full-time consultants as an additional incentive instrument.

Intrusions by central government actors into the hallowed domain of medical decision making were both more frequent and more visible during this period than ever before. But government actors neglected to explain the reasons for their activities. Without justifications of whatever sort, whether figures on expenditure or legal authority, intervention was blunted and had little impact on medical decison making. The failure of planning in the NHS reflects the limits of government power in a weakly institutionalized interventionist policy regime. In the face of central government's attempts to assert its authority over health care providers, decentralized units and the medical profession exercised their decision-making prerogatives with some impunity. This kind of contest over domains creates instability in an interventionist policy regime. It can be resolved by a return to a segmented order or by further clarifications of the principles and norms that justify state intervention. In the event, both of these options seemed to have been adopted by central government actors, and their coexistence structured evolving roles and relations in the NHS in the next decade.

The End of an Era: 1979–1982

It did not take long for all the relevant actors, governmental and professional, to realize that the 1974 reorganization of the NHS was unworkable. The immediately identifiable problems ranged from the high cost of the reorganization, which strained both human and capital resources, to the enormity of the new structure that had been created. With too many tiers and too many administrators, planning had deteriorated into administration. By 1976 another Royal Commission was set up to "consider in the interests both of the patients and of those who work in the National Health Service the best use and management of the financial and manpower resources of the National Health Service" (Ham 1982:30). The Merrison Commission Report was published in 1979, a few months before the Conservatives were elected. Shortly after taking office, the Thatcher government issued its own Consultative Document entitled *Patients First*, which recommended simplifying the administrative structure of the NHS, abolishing the Area Health Authorities, and streamlining and clarifying all functions. This document became the guide to another reorganization of the NHS, which took place in 1982.

Toward Interdependence Through General Management (1982–1989)

The purpose of the 1982 reorganization was to achieve efficiency by reducing administration and allowing even more delegation downward, a purpose that not only reflected the problems of the NHS but also captured the political spirit of the times. The new 192 DHAs that replaced the AHAs (the former area and district units were amalgamated) represented the spirit of localism symbolic of the Conservatives' manifesto pledge to decentralize the NHS (Klein 1983:135). A Labour government had undertaken many new cost control measures in the 1970s and had set up the 1979 Royal Commission that reorganized the NHS once more. But the Conservatives, once in office, were able to use Labour initiatives more forcefully to achieve their own objectives.

During the early years of this phase, the central government adopted a number of new instruments of control that protracted micromanagement. Among these were efficiency savings,[30] so-called Rayner scrutinies,[31] and performance indicators.[32] Program budgeting continued to be used in the planning process, but it became "more a tool for monitoring past expenditures than a mechanism for projecting future growth" (Ham 1982:131). In 1982 a new accountability review process was introduced as an extension of the planning system. These reviews allowed the DHSS to examine in considerable detail and on an annual basis the extent to which health authorities were pursuing DHSS policy guidelines and priorities.[33] The secretary of state was granted the power to use additional measures to enforce compliance, such as suspending health authorities, reducing their financial allocations, or conducting special inquiries into the operations of seemingly recalcitrant health authorities. These final-authority threats were rarely used, preempted by other methods of achieving mutually agreeable goals.[34] But they still functioned effectively as deterrents.

Besides reorganization, a second solution to the problem of lack of coordination among the several divisions in the NHS was to bring them all under a system of general management. The Griffiths Report of 1983 is the hallmark of this phase for the principles of management it laid out.[35] The report reiterated ideas that had already been expressed in a 1976 inquiry into the NHS, namely that many of the tasks performed by the DHSS should be devolved to local health authorities and that management throughout should be simplified and thereby strengthened. It diagnosed the central ailment of the NHS as "the lack of a clearly defined general management function throughout the NHS. By general management we mean the responsibility drawn together in one person, at different levels of the organization for planning, implementation and control of performance" (Griffiths 1983:11). The significance of the Griffiths Report for present purposes is that it clarified the principles of efficiency and effectiveness underpinning the new roles and relations that had been evolving among NHS actors in this era. It also expressed new bases of decision making. No longer was policy-making informed by the implicit dominance of medical authority or by the technicalities of administrative instruments; rather, it was guided by strategic objectives for the NHS constructed within the arena of central government offices. Thus, while it operationalized the principles and norms of an interventionist policy regime, the Griffiths Report also laid the foundation for yet another kind of policy regime.

Modifying Central Intervention

The Griffiths Report summarized central and local government relations succinctly: "The centre is still too involved in too many of the wrong things and too little involved in some that really matter. . . . The Units and Authorities are being swamped with directives without being given direction" (Griffiths 1983:12). It noted that the central government had lapsed into day-to-day management and needed to "prune many of its existing activities" (Griffiths 1983:15). And it recommended the establishment of a "small, strong general management body" within the DHSS, adding in parentheses "(and that is all that is necessary at the centre for the management of the NHS)" (Griffiths 1983:2). The main function of this body would be "to ensure that responsibility is pushed as far down the line as possible, i.e., to the point where action can be taken effectively" (Griffiths 1983:2). The Griffiths Committee may have thought it was promoting devolution, but ironically the result was increased central control. Implementation of the report's recommendations initiated a firmer framework of central government policy than had existed until then, and a more powerful system of centralized authority in the NHS. It established, finally, the hold of principles of efficiency and effectiveness toward which the NHS had been moving for more than a decade. But the instrumentalities of central control introduced by the report were less interventionist than the micromeasures used a few years before. In addition, this form of general management was more focused and less abstract than the macroplans of an earlier era. The implementation of general management in the NHS more successfully included the collective enterprise (management teams) that had been lacking in earlier macroplanning efforts.

The recommendation that a general manager head all management teams (including the new NHS Management Board at the Department of Health) was considered outrageous by the health authorities and their respective teams. Despite popular conceptions to the contrary, the Griffiths Committee was not posing the role of the generalist as over and above that of the expert, nor was it suggesting that general managers necessarily be recruited from outside the NHS.[36] It was more concerned that whoever occupied the position of manager be willing to assume responsibility.

A few months after the report was issued the DHSS sent a circular to all health authorities enjoining them to adopt the recommendations for general management. It took several years to complete the process from regional to district and finally unit (hospital) levels. In the end, fewer general managers were recruited from the private sector than had been anticipated, probably because of the low salaries. The overwhelming majority were already NHS administrators.

The introduction of general management immediately changed the modalities of decision making. The Griffiths Report was critical of consensual management for having led to "lowest common denominator decisions" and "long delays in the management process" (Griffiths 1983:17). On the surface, this observation was a critique of the top-down approach to detailed management that had characterized DHSS and local health authority relations in the past. In the same breath, however, the committee was expressing a plea for leadership, which the NHS lacked.[37] Since leadership necessarily rests on some form of hierarchy or centralization, especially when contrasted to the lack of leadership in consensus management, the committee implied the need for a stronger central government role in health care policy-making.

The Griffiths Committee addressed the issue of accountability within the NHS more directly, and in so doing, located the leadership it was searching for. It felt that the nascent accountability review process represented a "good, recent development which provides a powerful management tool" (Griffiths 1983:12). Following the committee's recommendation, the review process was extended to all units of management within the NHS, including hospitals and units within hospitals. Accountability review can be understood as a measure of central control, enabling the DHSS to enforce its priorities. As such it conforms to the ideals of good management. But accountability reviews are also measures for developing mutually acceptable goals. Because of the discussions and negotiations that take place during the reviews, the review process became a learning mechanism for the DHSS, enabling it to relax its "priorities" targets if health authorities were unable or unwilling to meet them. The Griffiths Committee saw the review process as a tool to facilitate the full functioning of general management within a tight budgetary system and a set of internal controls equipped to reduce the need for central, isolated measures of intervention, such as efficiency savings and national performance indicators. In this way the accountability review process provided a stronger central framework than the planning process of the previous phases. It facilitated delegation without micromanagement.

Deeper Intervention in Professional Domains

The Griffiths Report also made explicit recommendations regarding the role of clinicians, arguing that they should be involved "more closely in the management process [and] participate fully in decisions about priorities in the use of resources," and adding that these activities would be "consistent with clinical freedom for clinical practice" (Griffiths 1983:6). To encourage more involvement, the committee suggested that each hospital develop a management budget, whose dimensions would require clinician input about workload and service objectives. The members felt that such inclusion of clinicians was "so critical to effective management at local level" (Griffiths 1983:6) that they took the initiative to begin a study of six hospitals, in which clinicians were involved in the budget management process of both the hospital and its units and in which each clinician was given in addition an individual budget to manage.

The early reviews of these demonstration projects indicated problems, to be sure.[38] But there was enough continuing optimism at DHSS about the strategy that the Department of Health undertook the implementation of a revised version of budget management, called the Resource Management Initiative. The freshly created NHS Management Board in the Department of Health worked closely with the Joint Consultants Committee to implement the Resource Management Initiative at six new experimental sites and to undertake joint monitoring and evaluation that would also include representatives from the Central Consultants and Specialists Committee and the Royal Colleges. A preliminary evaluation was mixed but indicated that sufficient improvement had occurred to warrant continuing and expanding the Resource Management Initiative (CCSC 1989).

The overriding purpose of the Resource Management Initiative was to involve doctors in the management process so that they could become more aware of the financial implications of their medical decisions. The initiative enabled the NHS "to give a better service to its patients, by helping clinicians and other managers to make better informed judgements about how the resources they control can be used to the maximum affect" (DHSS 1986:2). This goal constituted the foundation of a major "cultural change" in health care (Buxton, Packwood, Keen 1989:12). The Resource Management Initiative placed much less emphasis on budgets per se than did its predecessor (management budgeting), and it concentrated more on the provision and dissemination of better information of both a financial and clinical nature. It was a collective process of information management—individual consultants assessed their workload and project needs and discussed them with their clinical director, who then discussed the division's activities with directors of other divisions at the hospital level. At each point discussions could include negotiations or the development of controls for overspending and rewards for saving. In general, hospitals adopted a policy of not demanding cuts in clinical activity but, wherever possible, of collapsing staff costs in order to control expenditures (CCSC 1989:12). The processes seemed to blend macro and micro measures of management.

The financial benefits proved minimal at best. But when the notion of benefit was expanded to include involvement of doctors in management, the overall results were more positive. One evaluation noted that "elements of the Resource Management process have firmly taken root at all sites. Particularly, at the sub-unit level, there has been a major change towards more pro-active management by service providers" (Buxton, Packwood, Keen 1989:18). It added the further important observation that "concerns from the medical profession about doctors in management have diminished" (Buxton, Packwood, Keen 1989:11). This report concluded "positively about the value of the management processes and organizational structures associated with RM [resource management]" (Buxton, Packwood, Keen 1989:18). In a similar vein, another evaluation noted that clinicians at most of the hospital sites were developing a "sense of ownership of the system" through their involvement (CCSC 1989:4). Both reports emphasized that for the potential of the Resource Management Initiative to be more fully realized, authority relations in the NHS should continue to be restructured such that "in decentralizing responsibility the [general manager] of the hospital has to be willing to devolve power" (Buxton, Packwood, Keen 1989:12). At the same time, "clear central leadership is needed to maintain cohesiveness and momentum" (Buxton, Packwood, Keen 1989:15).

Resource management has now become a major avenue for involving doctors in a broader set of social relations in health care. As has been noted throughout, past efforts to influence doctors have been circumscribed by the sanctity of clinical autonomy and have ceased before any boundary was approached. Traditionally, the provision of medical care in Britain has been ruled strictly by clinical autonomy. Agreeing to such freedom was one basis of the profession's acceptance of the NHS. Although doctors themselves find it difficult to articulate exactly what clinical autonomy means, it is generally understood to mean that their decisions on the treatment of individual patients are free from outside interference, most commonly from external organizations and institutions such as the government, but also from other doctors.[39] Beyond the self-regulation of British doctors through the General Medical Council,[40] clinical autonomy protected and isolated individual doctors within traditional authority relations.

But with the development of accountability reviews and other assessments and audits of clinical practice, clinical autonomy very gradually began to diminish in Britain. We might also point to the earlier RAWP process as one of the first steps in this movement toward greater clinical accountability. Insofar as the studies informing RAWP revealed vast inequities in medical care, outcomes, and expenditures across the country, questions were raised about the role of doctors in contributing to these differences.[41] But the power of clinical autonomy has been so sacrosanct in Britain that the government did not do anything directly to begin auditing clinical practices. Instead, it indirectly engineered more interest within the medical profession about medical audit. The mechanism of the shift was the powerful implicit threat to develop external controls unless the profession developed its own system. The profession responded positively. As one of its prominent members, Sir Raymond Hoffenberg, said: "the profession should welcome greater scrutiny of clinical competence, for only in this way will public confidence be maintained and the threat of external regulation avoided" (quoted in Ham and Hunter 1988:11). Indeed, in this dimension of professional/governmental relations, the acrimony that can accompany direct government intervention was largely avoided.

By the late 1980s the Royal College of Physicians accepted the challenge and offered to "undertake studies of selected and specific topics with a view to producing guidelines for clinical practice" (Hoffenberg 1989:8). Thus began an effort to enable the profession to recognize that its medical role necessarily included an understanding of the management of resources: "Ideally, review should include both clinical outcome and cost; unnecessarily extravagant practices used for some patients deprive others of their appropriate share" (Hoffenberg 1989:1).

Medical audits in Britain began as a simple form of peer review. There was no standard form for conducting the process. In some hospitals consultants selected cases either randomly or systematically for discussion; in other hospitals visiting teams of consultants analyzed either physician practices, cases, or activities. By 1989, however, the voluntary, completely intraprofessional quality of medical audit began to change. In its White Paper, *Working for*

Patients, the government announced that it would fund continuing development of medical audit by the Royal Colleges. More important, the White Paper delineated a role for management in working with the profession to further develop and conduct audits, and to initiate independent audits when necessary (Ministry of Health 1989e). Medical audits for general practitioners were also suggested. Throughout, the White Paper paid allegiance to the professional nature of audits, but it also noted that medical audits are an integral component of the management of resources. Henceforth, therefore, medical audit advisory committees would be established in each district and regional health authority, involving the relevant general managers. In the reorganized NHS that followed the 1989 White Paper, medical audits became a critical criterion in the allocation of contracts for doctors and hospitals.

In many ways, this era of management institutionalized the principles and norms of roles and relations characteristic of an interventionist policy regime. However, the tools of intervention were so qualitatively different from those used in earlier eras that they created a more cooperative working environment for intervention. General management is less intrusive than RAWP formula calculations, and peer-led accountability reviews are more acceptable than centrally determined performance indicators. The intervention that occurred in this era, then, paved the way for the possible emergence of a new policy regime, based more explicitly on accommodation, cooperation, and collaboration.

Back to a Social Contract for Health Care (1989–)

After ten years of Conservative government administration and rhetorical noises about making the NHS run more like a business, another major review of the NHS took place. It resulted in another reorganization—in fact, the most radical since the founding of the NHS. For the first time, functional as well as structural factors were affected, bringing about a more profound change in the principles and norms informing roles and relations within the NHS than any of the preceding reorganizations. Most important, the significance of central authority in the NHS has become more apparent to all health care actors. It is providing a stable reference point that enables actors to engage in a collective construction of new rules for health care provision.

Integrative Intergovernmental Relations

The 1989 White Paper, *Working for Patients*, proposed a devolution of responsibility. What took place can be seen as less a transfer than a sharing of tasks and accountabilities among the various units in the health care system. The NHS Management Executive and the NHS Policy Board, both in the Department of Health, have become clearer units of central control. The regional health authorities (RHAs) acquired most of the burden of deciding how to allocate funds to the districts, a task that had previously been centered in the DHSS. RHAs are now "expected to act on behalf of the Department in planning and managing services in their localities" (Ham 1991:21). However, the new rules of allocation are not reinstatements of separate domains of authority: RHAs essentially carry out central guidelines. Similarly, the devolution of decision making from regional to district health authorities and family health services authorities reflects a streamlined but still centralized authority structure within which decentralized units exercise contained discretion.

District Health Authorities

The 1989 White Paper, *Working for Patients*, offered the grounding for an important conceptual breakthrough in the roles and relations of NHS actors by changing the principles on which DHAs receive funds. It proposed that DHAs no longer be considered as providers of health care; they were to become purchasers instead. As of 1991 all DHAs are allocated budgets based not on their services but on the number of persons in their jurisdictions (capitation), adjusted for age (with a greater weighting for numbers of elderly), sex, and health status (measured by morbidity of resident population). These calculations replaced the RAWP formula for allocating funds. Within their allotted budgets DHAs decide what services to purchase. They must first assess the health needs of their residents, decide what types of services best meet these needs, and then (very importantly) decide with whom to form contracts for the provision of these services. Contracts are made with a variety of providers: general practitioners, community care facilities (which provide, for example, home care and day care for the chronically disabled or elderly), and hospitals in the public, private, or voluntary sectors. DHAs can contract with providers in their own or neighboring jurisdictional districts. Different kinds of contracts are made, depending on the services purchased: Block contracts for core services fund a given level of capacity (similar to American HMOs); cost and volume contracts specify a baseline of activity beyond which funding is assessed on cost per case (similar to a block grant); cost-per-case contracts are generally for elective procedures not covered by the previous two types of contracts (Ministry of Health 1989c:9–11).

The change to purchaser status has given DHAs considerable discretionary power, removing earlier intrusions from central government and establishing DHAs as "agencies which can challenge providers and hold them accountable for their performance" (Ham and Heginbotham 1991:6). However, DHAs are not completely independent actors in the decision-making process. They must obtain community input through regular meetings of local community boards, which include residents and local practitioners. At the same time, RHAs continue to perform several important functions: They provide considerable advice and assistance to DHAs in constructing contracts, and they are watchful that DHA activities implement not only community goals but also DHSS priorities and guidelines. In addition, RHA supervision facilitates standardization of decisions across districts; RHAs are a vehicle for information sharing as well as for encouraging districts to pool resources when appropriate.

One of several consequences of the change in DHA functions has resulted from the encouragement to pool resources. The overall number of DHAs has shrunk while the average size of their catchment populations, although varying from 250,000 to 750,000, has grown. Mergers between adjacent districts have occurred for a number of reasons: to achieve economies of scale, to reduce staff and administrative functions, to increase the financial leverage of DHAs against providers, and to increase competition among providers.[42] The initiatives for mergers came from the Department of Health, which continues to suggest the possibility of more, but they are undertaken fully consensually by DHAs themselves. At present there are 112 DHAs compared to 192 previously. Despite the enormous administrative changes that DHAs have undergone, it is estimated that their administrative expenditures have been kept at 0.5 to 1 percent of their budgets.

The new roles of DHAs created fledgling problems, from a need

for a new kind of expertise at local levels[43] to a need to reconcep-
tualize the relationship between jurisdictional boundaries and service provision. Yet another set of problems is imminent in a proposal to abolish RHAs by 1996 and fold their functions into the NHS
Management Executive. However, if DHAs in fact learn the rules of
collaborative behavior through their several consolidations and
joint purchasing arrangements, they may weather this administrative reorganization well. Further streamlining in the administrative structure of the NHS could, in fact, lead to greater coordination
between central and local levels. It could also, of course, create
fragmentation, especially among those DHAs that have not learned
or sufficiently institutionalized the principles and norms of collaborative roles and relations, especially with each other, if not
providers.

The social relations between local and central units of government have clearly changed. Because DHAs now have control over
allocating their own budgets and eventually over accruing savings
and thus determining to some small extent the size of their budgets,
they are in a less adversarial position with the central government.
The relationship between district and central levels, between, in
effect, purchaser and funder, is contractual. In fact, individual corporate contracts outline the "agreements through which the national agenda is taken forward . . . [and] the success criteria against
which [each DHA's] particular performance will be judged."[44] Collaboration is thereby being generated from the bottom up as well as
from the top down.

Self-governing Hospital Trusts

A similar transformation in financial and decision-making responsibilities occurred with hospitals. The 1989 White Paper charted a
transition in which hospitals would no longer receive funding
based on their operations but would instead become self-governing trusts, earning their own revenues based on the services they
provide. Ultimately, this is NHS money, for the most part, but the
rationale for the transfer of funds—granting hospitals complete
discretion over their resources—represents a fundamental change
in principle.

Any single hospital, group of hospitals, or group of hospital(s)
and community services can apply for self-governing trust status.[45]
There are specific eligibility criteria: provision of basic core and

other services; a board of directors with demonstrated management skills and senior professional staff, especially consultants, involved in management; a working system of medical audits; and financial viability (NHS 1990:3). Self-governing status offers hospitals much greater financial freedom than before. They "own" their own assets and so can acquire or dispose of assets as they see fit; they can borrow money and build up reserves; they are free to employ their own staffs at rates they negotiate; and they decide what services they will provide. These activities are governed by a "contractual" obligation to serve the public, for hospital trusts are still within the NHS. There is an implicit understanding among trusts that cost equals price. If a trust makes a profit, that money is plowed back into health care, according to decisions made by hospitals' governing boards. The relationship between self-governing trusts and the NHS as a whole is similar to that of general practitioners; both are independent contractors.

For its part, the DHSS acts as overseer without directly intervening in the operations of trusts. Two stipulations imposed by central government are restrictions on executive salaries and board member stipends and on eligibility for board membership (GPs, DHA employees, and so on, are not eligible). Trusts are accountable directly to the Department of Health (rather than to RHAs as before). They must provide information on their activities to the Department of Health on a quarterly basis (or monthly if the department wishes to increase monitoring). If the secretary of state decides to close a hospital or dissolve a trust, legal rights revert to the Department of Health or are transferred to another trust. In addition, the secretary of state retains "reserve powers" over hospital trusts, for use as necessary to "issue directions" or "institute inquiries" (Ministry of Health 1989b:7). The National Audit Office continues to audit the accounts of hospital trusts and has the right to request any information on financial arrangements and accounts, although in general, financial decisions are up to the trust and its board of directors. Trusts are required to display their accounts publicly once a year. Since the Department of Health is not itself a purchaser, however, health authorities and other purchasers who contract with self-governing hospital trusts engage in their own monitoring activities to assure that their money is being well spent. Individual hospitals decide whether or not to open routine meetings of the board of directors to the public or community health council representatives.

The 1989 White Paper suggested a system by which self-governing hospital trusts could develop contracts with both purchasers and other providers. Trusts contract with DHAs, independent GPs, specialists, nurses, private patients or their insurance companies or employers (there are Department of Health guidelines on the use of private financing), and other hospitals or community facilities with, for example, different technologies for diagnoses and services. Various indirect and market-based methods of accountability enter into hospital trust interactions with purchasers. For instance, DHAs and GPs may specify certain performance targets, such as waiting times or lengths of hospital stays, thus assuring quality in provision of services. Contracts may also specify that providers (hospitals) furnish purchasers (for example, DHAs) with patient satisfaction surveys and reports of actions taken to remedy complaints (Ministry of Health 1989b:11–12). In addition, hospital trusts are allowed to advertise their services, since these are the bases of revenues and contracts, but advertisements are subject to professional codes of conduct.[46] The principle of competition is expected to work in such a way that unviable hospitals can be identified. Where financial problems have arisen for hospitals, they have frequently been due to shifts in the purchasing patterns of DHAs. DHAs are no longer obligated to use district hospitals. They have in fact shopped around for better prices and found them elsewhere. These shifts have negatively affected urban hospitals, but they have also reduced past problems of redundancy in urban health care provision. The Department of Health has ultimate responsibility for deciding what to do with failing hospitals. Closures have occurred. Decisions to close only wards are up to individual hospital trusts; however, the Department of Health offers advice. Although trusts do not have to conduct consultations on their operational decisions, they are duty bound to inform purchasers ahead of time of major changes in provision.

The transition to self-governing trust status was expected to be gradual and, though voluntary, eventually to include all public hospitals in Britain. In fact, it has occurred quickly and smoothly. In 1994 only twenty-two NHS hospitals remained directly governed by their DHAs. The NHS Management Executive, acting through RHAs, takes an active role in supporting and guiding hospitals toward self-governing status.

In these early stages of the current reorganization in the NHS, the interrelationships among the various actors are several and complex. One layer consists of competition and bargaining among providers and between purchasers and providers. However, within another layer contractual arrangements among purchasers and providers in the public, private, and voluntary sectors induce more cooperative relations. The specific roles of central government actors are consultative and facilitative: to give advice and/or assistance, and to suggest additional collaborative networks. The central government does not intervene. Nor are central government actors particularly adamant about informing local actors of a major goal behind this reorganization: to improve the financial health of the NHS by making decisions about funding as efficient and effective as possible. The reorganization caused an unprecedented increase in total health care expenditures in Britain (see Chapter 6). But NHS officials are confident that cost control can be achieved.

The features of these current roles, relations, and decison-making modalities among state and local actors in the NHS are decidedly different from those that prevailed in earlier eras. The principle of separate rights and responsibilities that informed a segmented policy regime is not relevant to the kind of advisory functions that central government actors undertake in guiding local governments on the best purchases for their populations. Local actors, in turn, seek out the technical skills of those in central government. Nor do central government actors make any claims about the superiority of their knowledge, as they did within the earlier interventionist policy regime. Now they inform local actors of the decisions being made elsewhere, and they demonstrate alternative consequences of purchasing decisions, but they allow local actors to decide among the available options. These new principles and norms pertaining to roles, relations, and decision making are emergent. They evoke the characteristics of an integrative policy regime. At the same time, integration is pragmatic, yielding when necessary to the (re-) assertion of power by any set of actors. The best purchases remain those that maintain the economic health of DHAs and trusts. Thus, vestiges of segmented and interventionist policy regimes survive, but they do not detract from the turn toward flexible evaluation and decision making on needs and resources.

Integrative Professional–Governmental Relations

Hospital Consultants

Since the founding of the NHS, consultants have contracted with the NHS through regional hospital boards and later regional health authorities. The terms of the contracts were simple, stating what percentage of time the consultant would devote to NHS duties and with which hospital(s) s/he would be affiliated. The major sources of contention between consultants and the NHS had less to do with contracts or salaries, insofar as these were standard, than with the use of private beds in NHS hospitals for private-paying patients. This simplicity in consultants' contracts has changed, along with their accountabilities.

Consultants remain independent contractors, but now they sign agreements with hospital trusts. Trusts, in turn, have the freedom to develop their own contracts with the various staff members they employ. From having been accountable basically to their profession, consultants are now explicitly accountable to hospital general managers. Each general manager and each consultant works together to develop a job description that includes clinical and other duties, a schedule of hours and locations, participation in medical audit, out-of-hours responsibilities, budgetary and other management duties, and salaries (Ministry of Health 1989f:6). In addition, insofar as hospital trusts seek to maintain financial viability, they may require that consultants bring all or a specific portion of their private-paying patients to them. These job descriptions and terms of employment are reviewed annually by the two parties involved. Some consultants contract with more than one hospital. Some also contract with DHAs and/or GPs and/or community care trusts. Consultants may remain in the NHS superannuation scheme if they wish. They continue to be eligible for NHS distinction awards, but these are now paid by the employer (hospital trust). Because these contracts carry the possibility that consultants might become disengaged from their responsibilities to their hospital's management functions, the 1989 White Paper proposed modifying the criteria for distinction awards. The awards now reflect not only clinical skill but also "commitment to the management and development of the service" (Ministry of Health 1989a:44). The White Paper also proposed that award committees be headed by the chair of each RHA and that senior management as well as clinicians be involved in the award and promotion process. Awards are now reviewable every five years, with age limits and demonstrable contribution to management as criteria for the receipt of the higher awards (Ministry of Health 1989f:8–9).

General Practitioners

The 1989 White Paper introduced voluntary changes for GPs as well, expanding their managerial duties and promising to raise their professional status vis-à-vis consultants by giving them greater referral freedom. GPs are now offered the option of switching from an independent, capitation-based practice to inclusion in a GP practice budget scheme, called fundholding. Fundholding GPs have full control over their funds, deciding how to spend, what to buy, and whom, where, and how to treat. The number of patients on a GP's list is still the basis of each GP's income and represents the general medical care allowance for each GP. However, fundholding involves more than each GP's allowance, and these additional factors cannot be used to supplement the income of GPs. The funds are controlled not by individual GPs but by groups of practitioners; in fact, the scheme is intended to encourage group practices.[47] Despite vociferous opposition from the BMA, by 1994 approximately one-quarter of all GPs had formed fundholding groups. The proportion is expected to increase to one-half within the next few years.

Each GP fundholding budget includes a calculation for (1) typical hospital use, including inpatient care and use of diagnostic technology; (2) community care services (such as physical therapy); (3) staff costs, including fund managers (a new and required position), nurses, counsellors, and so on; and (4) purchase of equipment (computers for administration, medical technologies that enable GPs to provide more services themselves). These costs are estimated for the number of patients in the practices, weighted for age, sex, and morbidity.[48] There is a separate budget for drugs and prescription services. Fundholding GPs are free to contract with hospitals and other providers of services they do not offer, within the range of types of contracts (block, cost and volume, cost per case).[49] At first, most contracts with hospitals were made on a predetermined, fixed-cost, block basis (like the American DRGs), so that if hospital care exceeded the contracted amount, the hospitals had to absorb the loss. Recently, however, more GPs have begun to use cost-per-case purchasing, which allows them to specify the terms of treatment and to shop around for the best price. As a result of their entrepreneurial behavior, GP fundholders are being credited for demanding and receiving shorter hospital stays and reduced waiting times for elective surgeries.[50]

For each patient, GPs can decide whether they or some other provider in the public, private, or voluntary sector should provide the service, and what level of care is reasonable.[51] The role of the GP as the manager of an individual's total care is thereby reinforced. Insofar as GPs are both providers and purchasers of health care services, there is some indication that they may be performing more services themselves, including diagnostic testing and minor surgeries, rather than referring to specialists or hospital care. Concerns about underservicing are therefore being raised (Smedley et al. 1989:13). However, GPs have little general discretion over the use of any savings they manage to accrue; they must "plough back savings into their practices" (Ministry of Health 1989a:48). They have considerable substantive discretion, though, on how to do so (for example, whether to buy more mental health care or better office computers). Nevertheless, to control for abuse and assure that "money follows the patient" in this scheme, GPs are monitored by the family health services agencies (FHSA). Special budgetary reviews occur whenever GPs overspend,[52] but since all practices are reviewed every three years, problems of underspending can be investigated as well. RHAs and family practitioner committees conduct these budgetary reviews. Fundholding GP practices are also subject to statutory audits by the Audit Commission and the National Audit Office.

The mechanics of fundholding were less well articulated and, indeed, less well understood in the early stages than the other organizational changes taking place in the NHS. The first GPs who undertook the venture had to make up most of the rules as they went along (Glennerster, Matsaganis, Owen 1992:15). But they were given considerable flexibility as well as support, particularly from DHAs and FHSAs.[53]

As with the ventures in increased privatization (see Chapter 5), there is some concern about the consequences of market intrusions in GP behavior. Inequities in delivery and provision could result (both within and across practices). GPs may engage in "cream-skimming," shedding responsibility for the care of their more costly patients. GPs may also be so driven in their search for better prices as to ignore the comfort that comes from familiarity with local facilities. A study of the first year of fundholding found that none of these was occurring, but the sample size was small (ten practices) (Glennerster, Matsaganis, Owens 1992). Controlling adverse consequences of the market-based changes will depend on two factors. First, the central government must provide overall leadership, both itself and through its designated agents who monitor medical practices. Second, part of that leadership and the message it imparts must pertain to the broader goals of health care per se. One goal in institutionalizing this scheme was economic and has gone under the rubric of efficiency. Another goal was substantive and has been summarized by the term *effectiveness.* Although politicians and civil servants say they aim at value for money, they are only in the beginning phases of specifying the health care outcomes that are valued. Nevertheless, the task has begun and, interestingly, it is being conducted through the development of audits by the medical profession.

Medical/Clinical Audits

The 1989 White Paper offered a vague and descriptive definition of *audit*: "the systematic, critical analysis of the quality of medical care, including the procedures used for diagnosis and treatment, the use of resources and the resulting outcome and quality of life for the patient" (Ministry of Health 1989e:3). It offered no advice on how audits were to be conducted. Subsequent years brought considerable experimentation and eventually acceptance of audit as integral to the processes of health care. The various royal colleges and their faculties are developing their own auditing systems, which include procedures for meshing audits with performance reviews, and which are linked in some way with DHAs or hospital auditing activities. At the same time, various committees within DHAs and hospital and community trusts are engaged in auditing activities. For four years the NHS provided funds, totaling £221 million, to facilitate the initial phases of audits. As of 1994 the decentralized units are responsible for their own audit funding. For the most part, audits are now a necessary item in the budgets of all purchase contracts. The overriding assumption is that audits should be above all medically driven; however, the resource management implications of audits are a close secondary consideration.

Different methods of auditing pertain to GPs and consultants. Regarding GPs, all FHSAs, with whom GPs are affiliated, were required by the 1989 White Paper to set up medical audit advisory groups (MAAGs) "to direct, coordinate and monitor medical audit activities" within all GP practices (Humphrey and Barrow 1993:12). However, medical audit is not a contractual obligation for GPs, as it is for hospital consultants. The ability of GP practices to undertake auditing activities differs widely, depending on size and resources. Because it is understood that "formal audit is alien to the culture of general practice" (Humphrey and Barrow 1993:12), MAAGs are careful to ensure that auditing is, first and foremost, a process of simply collecting descriptive information. Only afterward does auditing include educative purposes, such as analyzing audit results and holding joint discussions between GPs and local medical committees. GP medical audit is circumscribed by rules of confidentiality and is not to be used to identify or correct poor practice. However, all FHSAs, to whom MAAGs report, have other mechanisms, mostly of an educational nature, to handle problematic GP practices. MAAGs are beginning to extend the range of medical audits undertaken and to strengthen the interfaces between GP medical practices (uni-professional and procedure-based activities) and clinical practices (management of care on a multiprofessional basis), as well as the interfaces between primary and secondary care.

The collaboration between royal colleges and hospitals in developing medical audits for the various specialties grew firmer in the 1990s.[54] Two types of expansion are now discernible: a closer connection between medical and clinical audit (that is, between uniprofessional and multiprofessional care) and a closer connection between audit and both resource management as well as peer review. What has changed, in other words, is the professional culture regarding audit. Audits within the medical specialties are moving from post facto descriptions to preemptive guidelines; they are now "established and accepted as a key method of setting and monitoring standards of clinical practice" (Stern and Brennan, no date, p. 9). The change has produced a new working definition of *audit*: a "systematic, quantified or qualitative comparison of specific medical practices against explicit current standards in order to identify opportunities to improve the quality of care to patients. This comparison is an on-going process" (Cambridge Training and Development, no date, p. 6).

All concerned are determined that audits for specialty care remain medically driven and that the professions have utmost and final determination. Managers are reminded that only peers can review doctors (Cambridge Training and Development, no date, p. 6). At the same time, doctors are reminded that reviews are not confidential matters. And they know that the "findings of audit will inform service development and purchasing" (Working Group 1993:1). This situation is unlike the roles and relations that pertained within either a segmented or an interventionist policy regime. Even though the medical profession retains its authority, practitioners are now more fully aware of their nonclinical roles as managers of scarce resources. Their participation in collective auditing processes and their frequent interactions with nonclinicians keep them apprised of the various criteria that enter into medical decision making. That decision making is no longer confined to a single predetermined paradigm supports the possibility that we are witnessing the emergence of an integrative policy regime.

Conclusion

Transitions in policy regimes in British health care have occurred through reorganization of the structural and administrative features of the NHS. Earlier reorganizations created new roles for government and professional actors that portended changing relations of power and increasing centralization. However, centralization and the interventionist policy regime it represents were frequently contradicted by the obduracy of traditional prerogatives. Local health authorities tended to interpret central directives as suggestions only and functioned as best they could (meaning as they saw fit). Doctors consistently held the upper hand in medical decisions, and their authority spilled over into extensive influence over resource allocation in the NHS. As a consequence of segmented relations, central government had to experiment with a variety of interventionist tools in its efforts to influence decision making in health care.

In many ways the most recent reorganization of the NHS can be seen as an accommodation to traditional domains. Vestiges of separate rights and responsibilities remain. And along with signs of returning centrifugal forces in the provision of health care, concerns are rising about the inequalities that inevitably accompany localisms. At the same time, there is an apparent resort to macromanagement, evident, for example, when the central government engages in advising and facilitating the providers of health care on alternative methods that conform to national priorities. Despite these indications, what must also be emphasized in the evolving social order of health care is the achievement of a new kind of central government authority—the ability to establish fundamental parameters for the NHS and see them adopted. The parameters are broad; they do not specify, as in the past, the acceptable wattage of light bulbs in hospital wards. Instead, they ask providers to consider all avenues of cost containment and provide examples of successful practices. An unusual convergence of past and present aspirations is occurring, echoing Bevan's early assessment that the NHS should be framed for a "maximum of decentralization to local bodies [and] a minimum of itemized central approval" (Klein 1983:49–50).

A main difference between now and the past is a closer integration of roles and relations among social actors. Both government actors at all levels and professional actors are less prone to air traditional prerogatives to avoid involvement. As a result, the NHS is no longer the bureaucratic and rigid social order it once was. Nor is it the paragon of the Conservatives' hopes for a return to market principles of organization. Along with a relaxation of past tensions has come a special focus on health care itself. Although economic and political factors continue to inform the dynamics of change in the NHS, a more inclusive understanding of health care underpins decision making. It appears not only in the development of medical audits, but also in the publications of central government (where organization charts have been replaced by health outcome indicators). These signs of change are subject to interpretation, but among the possibilities they suggest is the emergence of an integrative policy regime.

NOTES

1. I refrain from using the term *physician* in this chapter in favor of the more generic term *doctor* because in Britain a physician is commonly a type of specialist. When necessary I refer specifically to general practitioners or hospital consultants.

2. Krieger (1986) reaches a similar conclusion about the consequences of the Thatcher era in general for the role of the state.

3. The famous Beveridge report, published in 1942, called for social security "from the cradle to the grave." It was then Member of Parliament (later Prime Minister) Harold Wilson who used the quasi-religious imagery in 1956 (Allsop 1984:37).

4. A 1926 Royal Commission report first proposed "divorcing the medical

service entirely from the insurance system and recognizing it, along with all other public health activities, as a service to be supplied from the general public funds" (quoted in Forsyth 1966:1). GPs opposed the proposal and in the following decades honed their combative tactics should it arise again.

5. An initial proposal to set explicit financial controls, especially on the more profligate regional hospital boards, was modified and replaced by a ceiling on total expenditures, leaving to the hospital boards the task of deciding which services to reduce. As it turned out, decisions on these boards were dominated by doctors. Nonmedical members deferred to professional power in defining the terms of medical care within state-imposed ceilings.

6. See the discussion of this problem for a different set of policies in Ruggie (1984, Chapters 3 and 5).

7. The act in essence brought early forms of "private" insurance, such as Friendly Societies and Sick Clubs, under government regulation.

8. Local insurance committees, which dispensed GPs' payments, became coordinated under a General Medical Services Committee, whose area became contiguous with local authorities.

9. Although the terms *specialist* and *consultant* are used interchangeably, I refer to those specialists who have assumed some NHS duties as hospital consultants. There are many different kinds of physicians who are not GPs. Hospital consultants by now are the main group of non-GP physicians.

10. There are three grades of awards. "C" awards were commonly given to consultants after a few years of service. Most could expect eventual upgrading to "B" awards, but the "A" and especially the "A+" awards tended to favor consultants in teaching hospitals. The awards and promotions were decided entirely on an intraprofessional basis, and once obtained were held until retirement (Forsyth 1966:30). GPs have not been part of the award system.

11. Items whose costs and payments were constantly tinkered with were prescriptions, medical devices (such as eyeglasses), dental services, and private beds in hospitals (pay beds). Throughout the years the financial adjustments made on these items "caused controversy disproportionate to the sum raised" (Parry 1986:162).

12. Hoping to rejuvenate Britain by creating an ethos of efficiency, Harold Macmillan, a Conservative prime minister, introduced planning into a wide range of government activities (cf. Beer 1982). Macmillan offered an unusual philosophy for a Conservative. Before becoming prime minister he wrote a book, *The Middle Way*, "expounding the case for economic efficiency and rational social organisation" through planning, not competition (Klein 1983:64). That planning was introduced under a Conservative government may well have eased its acceptability. A White Paper on public expenditure recommended that government engage in forecasting capital expenditures in all sectors of the economy. (The White Paper is cited by Ashford [1981:106] as 1960, Cmnd. 1203.) It was followed by a major inquiry into the problem of planning public expenditure, resulting in the 1961 Plowden Report. Despite its failure to change the way the Treasury operated, for our purposes the Plowden Report marked the beginning of an era of technocratic rationalism in government, in which objective measures of performance were used to justify decisions taken by all NHS actors. The Plowden Report "paved the way for the separation of the civil service from

the Treasury" by suggesting that the civil service (as well as nationalized industries themselves) conduct better cost analyses so as to be more accountable to
the Treasury for current and future (planned) expenditures (Ashford 1981:70,
107). In the case of health care the Plowden recommendations meant that the
Ministry of Health needed to understand better and to justify more concretely
the bases of expenditures. However, the central government continued to shun
this task, leaving the determination of internal expenditures up to the providers
and local health authorities. The Plowden Committee understood that control
of public expenditures necessitated more precise measures of economic variables and economic behavior. It called for more cost–benefit analysis, better
accounting, and more efficient budgeting. The enthusiasm for planning expenditures created many new government units and instruments. These included
the National Economic Development Council; Programme Analysis Review;
and Planning, Programming, and Budgeting (Heclo and Wildavsky 1974). Soon
after the Plowden Report was published in 1961, a new method of budgetary
allocation, the Public Expenditure Survey Committee, was set up in the Treasury (and still exists); it began to systematize the previously ad hoc format of
budgetary allocations. Despite these additions to government activities, deciding the budgets of the various ministries has remained essentially a process of
political negotiation between the Treasury and the ministries.

13. Ham lists the stated purposes of reorganization as unification of the tripartite system, coordination of health and welfare services, and better management of the system as a whole (1982:27–28). Allsop discusses five: administrative unification, centralization and priorities, management, planning, and
democratic accountability (1984:61–68). Although hailed as a product of the era
of "faith in the ability of organizational change to promote greater efficiency
and effectiveness" (Klein 1984:90) and the "zenith of the managerialist phase"
(Allsop 1984:60), the need for unification had long been suggested. The original
tripartite structure had been a necessary concession to political and historic
patterns of authority. Despite the problems it entailed, especially regarding
intergovernmental relations, no one recommended altering it while the NHS
was still in its formative stages. But by the early 1960s the need for change was
becoming clearer to all involved, including local authorities themselves. As
early as 1962 the medical profession, reporting through the Porritt Commission, also voiced its approval of a unified health service.

14. My inconsistency in using the terms *Ministry of Health, Department of
Health, Department of Health and Social Services* (and later, NHS *Management
Executive*), and so on, reflects historical variations in the names used by the
government itself and in the literature. At all times I apply the term common
for the period. The structure described here is for England only. Some minor
differences characterized the reorganized NHS in Wales, Scotland, and Northern
Ireland.

15. The RHAs took over from the regional hospital boards. Each RHA had
twenty members, all appointed by the secretary of state for the Department of
Health and Social Security, and all unpaid except for the chair, who received a
part-time salary. These RHAs were to develop ten-year "strategic" plans and to
work with the DHSS, assume its national priorities, and interpret these in relation to the different areas within each region.

16. Their members were appointed by RHAs, local authorities, and nonmedical and nursing staff (Ham 1982:29). They were to prepare three-year "operational" plans in consultation with the RHAs. In most localities except London, AHAs were made coterminous with local authorities, which provided personal social services, so as to coordinate joint planning and joint provision of health and welfare services.

17. DHAs were administered by management teams and advised by Community Health Councils. These councils (there were about 200 in England) were to incorporate participatory democracy so as to represent "consumer" interest at the most local level. There were about 200 Health Councils in England. Eventually, the DHAs prepared five-year strategic plans as well.

18. The calculation of need was based on demographic factors, mortality rates, and hospital beds. The next step in using the RAWP formula—applying it to reallocating resources—was less technical. In fact, the original working party did not regard an examination of the link between measures of need and resource allocation as part of its charge; it did not suggest what services should be used or what service planning should be conducted (Paton 1985:7). Allocation figures were based less on the RAWP formula (because these measured need) than on previous years' expenditures. Combining the need and allocation data yielded rough, long-term (ten-year) reallocation targets for the fourteen regions. To ease the transition toward a situation in which the richer regions would lose funding, incremental short-term targets were also set.

19. The formula assumed more than it delivered. It assumed that calculation of need could determine the allocation of resources, that reallocated resources could achieve improved services, and that improved services could lead to reduced inequalities in health outcome. However, no further attention was given to these inequalities.

20. Because the goal was to encourage collaboration, the joint-care programs were not always well incorporated into or reflective of larger plans for the development of services (Allsop 1984:114).

21. These planning guides outlined how local health authorities should review existing services and determine needs and goals; select among appropriate means available; implement, monitor, and evaluate results and progress; and consult with interested parties throughout—specifically, community health councils, family practitioner committees, area advisory committees, joint staff consultative committees, and most important, local social service authorities with whom health service provision was to be coordinated. Issued in 1976, *The NHS Planning System* laid out the planning methodology, and *Priorities for Health and Personal Social Services in England* presented central government goals for greater attention to dependent groups. The DHSS was very specific about the changes expected, indicating the importance of using program budgeting as a "framework for linking policies with resources, thus enabling priority decisions to be made within an overall strategy" (Ham 1982:129). Targets for annual growth rates for all local health and personal social services incorporated the goal of shoring up the Cinderella services.

22. The main noncentral government units affected by the hospital plan were the fourteen regional hospital boards, which were charged with the task of developing and overseeing the implementation of the plans. Most of the

members of these boards were selected by the Ministry of Health, so that the friction between the two levels could be kept under control. When conflicts in perceptions did occur, they tended to reflect and reinforce the semiautonomous nature of regional hospital boards.

23. The estimated catchment of 100,000 to 150,000 persons in the original plan was doubled to 200,000 to 300,000 by the time the plan made its way through the medical community and was revised again in the mid-1960s. This increase reflected the importance of large-scale operations to the medical profession.

24. The report on district general hospitals published in 1969 reiterated the importance of large hospitals for the efficient delivery of services. With doctors comprising twelve of the eighteen members of the committee and with the report also emphasizing the importance of specialists working in concert with adequate support staff, it was transparent whose definition of efficiency held currency.

25. For one, it recommended grouping doctors into "Firm and Division" positions. Furthermore, representatives of all the specialty divisions were to sit on newly created medical executive committees. These committees were intended to revamp and upgrade already existing medical advisory committees and were to make decisions on the allocation of all resources in hospitals, from the use of beds to the dispensation of treatments. The report also recommended special training for the chairs of the hospital medical executive committees as well as for those filling the new positions of administrative medical officers, whose jobs were more focused on obtaining the information needed to make administrative, not clinical, decisions. The report sketched the overall framework of these positions without specifying the roles and functions in detail. The Cogwheel initiatives can be thought of as preceptors of the business orientation in later stages.

26. By implication the idea of peer review was articulated, along with the notion that it is individuals who make mistakes and less so professional groups acting in concert. It was a bold insertion into the debate; however, the time was not ripe for its germination.

27. It is noteworthy that an earlier attempt to instill a managerial style into the activities of nurses proved more successful. Following the recommendations of the Salmon Report, a division between nurse managers and nurse practitioners established the importance of management as a specialist function in its own right. The Salmon Report has been criticized for being overly concerned with managerial changes in nursing to the detriment of clinical changes, but it prepared the nursing profession for its increased role in decision making following the 1974 reorganization (Allsop 1984:59).

28. The introduction of team management was another effort on the part of central government to flex its managerial muscles. In contrast to the initially advisory nature of changes introduced in the planning process for decentralized health authorities, the central government was from the outset much more prescriptive about the changes it expected in management in all spheres of the NHS. The 1972 Grey Book and the DHSS planning manual were insistent about the style of organization yet vague about the function of the management teams. The teams were to operate on the basis of consensus; they were not to "manage" as such, but to review services, propose plans, and monitor and coordinate

policy implementation (Klein 1983:86). Within these guidelines management teams could choose which specific items they wished to address. Although the items covered the full range of health care issues, by far the majority were of a routine or informational nature (Klein 1983:96) and focused on hospital matters (Schulz and Harrison 1984). Management teams had decision-making powers, and their decisions were directly transmitted to, and usually fully accepted by, the relevant branch (district, area, or regional) of health authority. Schulz and Harrison (1984:664) report that only rarely were the teams in their study unable to come to an agreement. Since decisions were based on consensus, there was little reason for health authorities not to accept them. Indeed, consensus made difficult decisions more palatable. Thus, a general management function, which was to become the core of the following phase, was introduced into the NHS as another mechanism through which central government could exercise a measure of control over decision making in the NHS.

29. Medical dominance was not always obvious to team members, because it was not overtly present in the political or negotiating process (Schulz and Harrison 1984:672–74). It appeared only in the outcome of decisions or in the endurance of traditional patterns of health care provision. For instance, insofar as the most important task of the district management team was recommending how the budget should be allocated, the continuing increase in hospital-based services revealed where power was concentrated. Studies of decision-making styles found little effort among the district management teams to evaluate services or improve their effectiveness, with the result that decisions tended to be more reactive than proactive, reflecting the interests of the status quo (Schulz and Harrison 1984:667).

30. These were the specific percentages of current annual spending that the central government expected local authorities to save; in other words, they were explicit figures of expected expenditure cuts. Within a few years they were replaced by cost improvement programs, which were less directive in that health authorities themselves indicated how they intended to become more efficient and generate savings (Ham 1982:48).

31. These are short, intensive studies of specific items (such as transport services, recruitment advertising, the collection of payments), which indicated where efficiency could be improved and money saved. A controversial consequence of one Rayner scrutiny study was selling property that had been used to house NHS staff (Ham 1982:49).

32. These presented statistical information on clinical services, finance, manpower, and management of capital in all hospitals and health authorities, providing a basis of comparison for the units. The data were intended to stimulate further investigation of the reasons for the differences (Ham 1982:49).

33. The process was initiated after the House of Commons Public Accounts Committee complained about the lack of DHSS control over the NHS (Ham 1982:71). The review process was conducted in two phases: first, DHSS and cabinet representatives assessed regional developments, and then the RHAs assessed district activities.

34. For instance, it became more common for civil servants at the DHSS and officers at the health authority units to exchange posts for a limited period of time, enabling cross-fertilization of perceptions and ideas.

35. For a study of the Griffiths era, see Harrison et al. (1992).

36. Given the private-sector backgrounds of the committee members and their sense that the similarities between NHS management and business management are more important than the fact that the NHS is not concerned with the profit motive, they no doubt assumed that some general managers could come from the private sector. Twelve of the fourteen regional general managers first recruited were from within the NHS. In all, only 10.5 percent of the total general managers appointed by 1985 came from the private sector. Also, only 10 percent were clinicians—medical or nursing officers.

37. "Absence of this general management support means that there is no driving force seeking and accepting direct and personal responsibility for developing management plans, securing their implementation and monitoring actual achievement" (Griffiths 1983:12). And on the next page, "the presence of a general management function would be enormously important in . . . providing the necessary leadership to capitalise on the existing levels of dedication and expertise among NHS staff of all disciplines, and to stimulate initiative, urgency and vitality" (Griffiths 1983:13). The words echo Weber's concept of charismatic authority as much as bureaucratic authority.

38. The problems were both technological (the computer systems were complicated and the utility of their programs was limited because based on limited information) and social (clinicians had not been sufficiently involved in the initial information gathering that went into the programming).

39. Citing a number of studies, Harrison and Schulz (1989:199) delineate four kinds of claims to autonomy: the right to independent practice, the right to refuse an individual patient, the responsibility to lead and coordinate other health professions, and the overarching primacy of medical knowledge.

40. One study (Ham and Hunter 1988) concluded that the accountability of doctors through complaints and disciplinary procedures is extremely limited.

41. Studies being conducted in the United States about variations in clinical practices and medical outcomes appeared in British journals and may have been influential. Wennberg's studies (for example, Wennberg and Gittlesohn 1973) are particularly noteworthy. The director of research at the Royal College of Physicians makes several references to the American literature in his book on medical audit (Hopkins 1990).

42. Joint purchasing between DHAs varies from informal arrangements (perhaps for such specific items as nursing homes) to formal consolidation as consortia or agencies. DHA purchasing agencies are similar to American health alliances that purchase insurance (in effect in some states, see Chapter 4). Some DHAs conduct joint purchasing with family health service agencies (FHSAs). This too will increase if a proposal proceeds to fold FHSAs into DHAs in 1996.

43. District general management functions now concentrate on purchasing contracts, some of which are exceedingly detailed (for example, a contract to purchase X number of Caesarean-sections with hospital Y; another for B number of physical therapy session with community facility C).

44. NHS Chief Executive. Draft Letter: "Priorities and Planning Guidelines for the NHS: 1995–96." 13 May 1994:1.

45. Mergers have occurred among trusts as well, primarily for market-based reasons, such as avoiding duplication. A similar transition to trust status is

occurring among community care providers, in some cases among themselves, in others as part of a hospital-based trust. For example, day care and home help service providers may form a trust, or a physicial therapist group may join a hospital trust. Whether incorporated or not, community care providers now contract with GPs, DHAs, and other purchasers of their services.

46. Since corporate governance is new behavior for hospitals, the NHS Executive has constructed a code of practice based on what private-sector companies do.

47. Individual GPs can have no more than 2,000 patients on their list. The initial minimum for fundholding status was high (11,000 patients) in order to encourage teams of GPs. It was reduced to 7,000, so that a minimum of three GPs must collaborate to form a fundholding practice. There is no stipulation for maximum size of these fundholding practices; at present, the range is from 5,000 to 22,000 patients. In all, there are about 2,000 fundholding practices involving about 6,000 GPs.

48. These calculations evolved as the experiment progressed. In the first wave of fundholding, budgets were based on historic patterns of service use, a system that tended to reward high spenders and discouraged low spenders from joining.

49. Because purchasing by GP fundholders parallels that of DHAs, the latter exclude that portion of the population served by GP fundholders from their own calculations. GPs and DHAs keep each other informed of their purchasing decisions.

50. Some fundholders have exercised their power of exit from inefficient local facilities. Early reports indicated patient satisfaction with these practices, even though improvements in service required, for instance, longer travel distances (Glennerster, Matsaganis, Owens 1992:27). In their survey Glennerster, Matsaganis, and Owens did not find any cases in which reduced waiting lists for fundholders created inequities for patients of nonfundholding GPs. Instead, nonfundholding GPs frequently picked up on the competitive spirit and made their own demands for shorter waiting times (Glennerster, Matsaganis, Owens 1992:31).

51. Level of care includes use of prescription drugs: A separate working paper addressed this role of GPs and offered suggestions for cost control (Ministry of Health 1989d). Once registered with a GP, patients have no freedom of choice of provider. They can, however, switch GPs.

52. Practices that overspend in excess of 5 percent for two years in succession may lose their right to participate in fundholding (Ministry of Health 1989d:13–14).

53. For example, because GPs were concerned about being "bankrupted" by very expensive patients, most DHAs agreed to pick up the bill for episodes over and above £5,000 (Glennerster, Matsaganis, Owens 1992:10).

54. In 1992 it was estimated (and acknowledged to be an underestimate) that more than 3,000 specialty groups were participating in audits, involving 70–80 percent of doctors; that approximately 2,800 projects were multidisciplinary; and that 310 cut across the primary/secondary interface (Stern and Brennan, no date:10).

Chapter Three

Canada

In the late 1980s the Canadian health care system experienced a brief period of acclaim (most notably in the United States). It had become a model of the "third way" in organizing health care—exhibiting neither the "socialized" qualities of the British system nor the excesses of private enterprise and lack of central control endemic to the United States. Canada's system permits many practices characteristic of private medicine, such as consumer choice of physician and fee-for-service remuneration. However, the government exercises considerable financial control in, for instance, global budgeting of physician payment and hospital costs. In retrospect, Canada's progress through the stages of development in its health insurance system seems smooth—the implementation of legislation brought little change for either patients or physicians aside from the method of payment. Recently, however, complaints have increased about many aspects of the delivery system, particularly the problems of longer waits for elective surgeries and less personalized physician care. These shortcomings have created an apparent disenchantment with the Canadian model, on both sides of the border. However, although Canadians may be searching for improvements in their system, they have no intention of radically transforming it.

The forces that were instrumental in creating the Canadian health insurance system, and that forged compromises on both intergovernmental and physician-related issues, are the same ones underlying its current travails. The central feature of the Canadian health care system, which both restricts and energizes its evolution, past and present, is federalism. It has several dimensions when applied to health care. Besides the conventional meaning in which federalism defines the formal relations between the provinces and the central government, it represents broader processes of tension and compromise between centrifugal and centripetal political forces. Comparable processes are evident in professional–governmental relations, where the disjuncture includes discord and accommodation between private provision and public funding. Although it is consistent with the pluralist approach, federalism offers important additional considerations about the roles and relations among interest groups and government actors, and it thereby suggests alternative formulations. Pluralist theory emphasizes that interest groups are the stimulus to which governments respond; interest groups are the real source of political authority. Federalist theorists agree in principle but note that powerful interest groups may create decentralizing and divisive social currents that destabilize political order. Similarly, weak professional organizations can precipitate centripetal forces, leading to greater centralization in decision making. I use the insights of federalist theory heuristically to investigate the roles and relations among medical and government actors in the development of health policy in Canada. Federalism is a multidimensional and dynamic process, embodying shifting balances of power. It describes different configurations of power among centralized and decentralized actors, as well as different avenues of change in social relations. The form of federalism in any given era appears in the extant policy regime organizing health care.

The Canadian constitution—the British North American (BNA) Act of 1867—established a clear jurisdictional division in the field of health care by splitting responsibility between the federal and provincial governments. It specified that the federal government would provide medical care for the military and naval services (Section 91:7) and establish, maintain, and quarantine marine hospitals (Section 91:11). It granted to the provinces not only specific jurisdiction over the establishment, maintenance, and management of hospitals, asylums, and charities other than marine hospitals (Section 92:7), but also, more generally, specific jurisdiction over "all matters of a merely local or private nature in the province" (Section 92:16) (Mahler 1987:86). This clear foundation of segmented roles and relations ruled health care until the 1930s. The jurisdictional issue itself need not have been problematical, and in fact did not raise any difficulties for decades, were it not for the accompanying constitutional provisions for fiscal powers. The federal government alone has the power to levy direct taxes (for example, on income); the provincial governments can levy only indirect taxes (for example, on sales). Furthermore, when fiscal powers and jurisdictional divisions collide, as they are bound to, the federal government has at its disposal one further constitutional prerogative: the power to disallow provincial legislation.

In liberal democracies the exercise of central government authority is commonly a second-order event, arising from strains in a separation of domains. In Canada the conditions under which the federal government can legitimately exercise its power of disallowance are not constitutionally specified and must be interpreted. And interpretations vary with time and politics. Federalism empowered the central government in the early years of the fledgling Dominion; a period (approximately from 1890 to 1940) followed in which a provincial-rights movement dominated politics; and this was followed by a return to a more centralized version of federalism (Russell 1990:40). But centralization has been uncertain, marked by several swings in power, all of which have been accompanied by crises—in constitutional interpretation, in governmental relations, and, in the case under study here, in the social relations of health care.

Through investigating how health policy reflects prevailing interpretations of federalism, I will also be asking whether federalism is a constraint on policy development, whether it provides opportunities for policy innovation, or both. The tenets of A. V. Dicey's argument that federalism gives rise to weak, conservative, and legalistic government remain the bases of criticisms (Gray 1991:10–11). They point to institutional and structural obstacles and restrictions, proliferated by large numbers of access points capable of preventing the extension of central government activity and the development of legislation promoting social change. In recent years a revisionist interpretation has argued that the large number of access points in federal systems can actually multiply overall government activism, witness the expansion in the 1960s in Canadian federal government involvement in several social policy fields. Some revisionists argue that "such expansionist activities have not offset the restrictionist side of federalism generally" (Banting 1987:41). Others highlight the "interplay between the configuration of interests in the health field and the political complexion of Canadian federalism at particular points in time" (Tuohy 1986:404).

The stages in Canada's health policy development can be captured by the organizing principles and norms of prevailing policy regimes. I discuss three broad phases in the development of health policy in Canada. In the first a number of forward-looking government actors tested constitutional inconsistencies regarding the role of the federal government in health care. However, in all cases the system of separate domains prevailed and reinforced health care as a provincial responsibility. Nevertheless, funding concerns continued to necessitate a stronger role for the federal government, an expansion that was supported by the medical profession. In a second phase the provinces allowed the federal government to assist them financially in their efforts to initiate hospital insurance. However, federal actors used their role more broadly. An interventionist policy regime thus developed alongside a segmented one. More complete institutionalization of an interventionist policy regime appeared with the development of insurance for medical care. Struggles by the medical profession to offset government intervention created a politics of contention that has continued to punctuate professional and governmental relations to this day. However, the legislative achievements of health policy in Canada and the ability of the federal government to uphold them have created unusual stability, allowing for more experimentation with alternative roles, relations, and modes of decision making. Recent developments, based on more accommodative, cooperative, and collaborative forms of provision and delivery, suggest the possible emergence of an integrative policy regime.

Preparatory Steps:
Testing the Dynamics of Federalism (–1948)

At the time of confederation (1867), health care in Canada was basically a private matter. Individuals relied on their own resources to purchase services, and hospitals were administered and financed by private charities and religious organizations. The constitutional division of jurisdictional responsibility in the BNA Act did not affect the status quo in health care delivery, nor did the creation of the Dominion alter the ongoing development of private insurance. As a result, by the time of World War II, health care provision and financing in Canada closely resembled the American counterpart. Just as groups in the United States were experimenting with prepaid plans, so too were Canadian reformers trying to expand beyond the indemnity principle of commercial insurance.[1] In addition, a number of politicians, primarily from the western provinces, were sufficiently impressed with the British experiment in national health insurance (1911) to call for similar actions by provinces (but not, it should be noted, by the federal government). They advanced little beyond setting up a few provincial commissions of inquiry and initiating provincial parliamentary debates, which kept the issue of public health insurance alive in the eyes of both politicians and the public.

Segmented Government

The constitutionality of a federal government role in health care provision was not questioned until 1935. A Conservative prime minister, R. B. Bennett, struggling for political survival, introduced legislation for a nationwide Employment and Social Insurance Act, which included a proposal for health benefits. The program was to be financed by a direct federal premium levied on all taxpayers, initiating greater federal government involvement in social policy.[2] In the first of many such responses, the province of Ontario challenged the federal initiative, and the Supreme Court of Canada agreed that the federal government's legislation exceeded its constitutional boundaries. Because these events uprooted a number of political problems and left them all unsolved, in 1937 the federal government, now under the progressive, Liberal Party leadership of

Mackenzie King, appointed its first major Royal Commission on Dominion–Provincial Relations (the Rowell–Sirois Commission). Its focus was the division of authority for social policy.

Defining a Federal Role

Reporting in 1940, the commission clearly reasserted that while old-age security and unemployment insurance fell under federal jurisdiction, workmen's compensation and health insurance were constitutionally provincial responsibilities. It recognized, however, the accompanying problems posed by the constitutional limits on provincial fiscal powers. It recommended that compromises and constitutional amendments be considered to enable national solutions to the financial problems incurred by provinces as they attempted to develop health insurance. It specifically rejected the use of conditional federal grants-in-aid to the provinces for health care programs.[3] But it noted that those provinces (read: the poorer provinces) wishing to establish health insurance plans more in line with innovations in other provinces (richer ones) could entrust the federal government with the collection of premiums, "delegat[ing] to the Dominion the authority to institute such a scheme . . . rigidity in the matter of jurisdiction should be avoided" (quoted in Taylor 1978:12). The commission's interpretation of federal relations represented a threshold in the pendulum of shifting power. The report legitimized a new, albeit secondary, role for the federal government in enabling the provinces to expand public-sector health care. Thus, while conforming to the principles of separate domains, it articulated a federal responsibility that became a foot in the door to a change in policy regimes.

The federal government role outlined in the report was not as far-reaching as the prime minister had envisioned. He nevertheless continued to advance his social policy goals. During World War II, King and his energetic minister of pensions and national health, Ian Mackenzie, felt that the time might be right to introduce wartime measures on unemployment and health insurance. The cabinet did not endorse these proposals because of the constitutional issues involved. So King sidestepped normal politics and proceeded on his own to gather support from provincial governments, professional medical associations, and consumer groups (including labor and farm groups). He set up a broadly representative advisory committee on health insurance, which recommended that conditional grants-in-aid were "the only feasible method of enabling provinces to introduce the proposed program" (Taylor 1990:48). The political debate that followed was influenced by support from several key private-sector organizations, including the Canadian Medical Association (CMA), the Canadian Hospital Association, and the Canadian Life Insurance Association (CLIA). They all agreed with the merits of a federal role in funding assistance to the provinces.

Elaborating the Federal Role

The task of actually constructing agreement on the necessary constitutional modifications and the political implications of a new fiscal relationship in public-sector health care was taken up by a federal/provincial conference.[4] An election delayed the conference, and its preparations were further dampened by the creation of a new Department of Health and Welfare with a new minister of health less committed than his predecessor to the degree of federal intervention that would be necessary to realize pending proposals for public health insurance. The Dominion/Provincial Conference on Post-War Reconstruction finally held in 1945 considered a wide range of social insurance measures. The health care components were toned down from earlier versions but were still far-reaching. There were four main items: (1) a planning and organization grant from the federal government to enable each province to establish a health insurance system; (2) a cost-sharing program to enable each province to implement a health insurance system; (3) a series of health promotion grants to all provinces; and (4) financial assistance for hospital construction.

These recommendations themselves were acceptable enough to all the conference participants, but the federal government's sweeping proposals for acquiring the funds it would reapportion to the provinces were not because of the expanded fiscal power that would accrue to the federal government.[5] Most important, the premier of Ontario voiced his disapproval of a large federal subsidy and stated his preference that each province collect its own taxes for its own health insurance expenditures. Quebec maintained a remote attitude throughout, expressing typical antipathy toward federal infringement on provincial prerogatives. Only Saskatchewan, which was already at the vanguard of health care planning, agreed fully with the federal proposals and asked only for a greater federal role in equalization of resources and in cost sharing. Manitoba was also enthusiastic, and eventually Alberta joined its prairie neighbors. With only one-third of the provinces in support and the rest unable to reach a mutually agreeable accommodation, the postconference committee put the proposals on hold. Government actors at all levels had mobilized a semblance of unity among their disparate interests with regard to health care financing—albeit a unity that was neither unquestionable nor solid. But powerful decentralizing forces remained. The federal government could not at this time impose even a tenuous conformity on the provinces.[6]

Yet, in this circuitous but typically Canadian way, the groundwork was laid for an expansion in public-sector health insurance.[7] What seemed at the time like an anticlimax actually marked the onset of a clearer understanding between the provinces and the federal government about what each would do in the development of health care. It was a demarcation of responsibilities that reinforced the ruling principles and norms of a segmented policy regime. But at the same time, it represented progress in expressing the involvement of government in general and the federal government in particular in health care. The federal government would act as grantor to the provinces, and through its facilitative funding would become a partner with the provinces in public-sector provision of health care. The key to developments in the following decades rests on the capacity of the federal government to use, occasionally and ingeniously, its fiscal role to be a leader as well as a facilitator.

Segmentation Between Profession and Government

In all phases of its history the medical profession in Canada has differed in significant ways from both its British and American counterparts. Unlike in the United States, general practitioners (GPs) in Canada have always been and remain central to health care provision.[8] And unlike the split between GPs and specialists that defined the early years of organized medicine in Britain and later plagued medical and administrative coherence in the NHS, intraprofessional ties have been firmer in Canada. Canadian doctors developed strong self-regulatory powers earlier than their counterparts in Britain or the United States, exercising control over licensure and fee setting through their provincial associations. The CMA, established in 1867, reinforced the cohesiveness of doctors through its code of ethics, which contained important clauses on solidarity in maintaining standard forms and amounts of remuneration.[9] Its insistence on fee-for-service as the basis of remuneration brought organized medicine in Canada into close alignment with its American counterpart. Indeed, maintaining fee-for-service reimbursement became a cornerstone of medical politics in Canada.

Government as Payer

The main difference between Canadian and American organized medicine is the former's consistently more favorable view of the role of government in health care. From early on, government support was recognized as "an important adjunct" in the provision of care, and government regulation was considered central to "the maintenance of an autonomous medical profession" (Naylor 1986:15). During the Depression the profession was favorably disposed to a government role in financing health care because of the accumulation of unpaid doctors' bills. The CMA lobbied provincial governments for funding assistance for indigent care. It even approached the federal government, where it was reminded of the constitution's delimitations.

Provincial governments in western Canada were more responsive to physicians' appeals. Saskatchewan expanded its salaried "municipal doctor system," and through its Relief Commission extended grants to doctors practicing in certain relief areas. Because of these cooperative relations, Saskatchewan's medical association in 1933 was one of the first to endorse the principle of public health insurance.[10] In several provinces, including Ontario, governments and medical associations came to agreements on subsidizing physicians for services rendered to the indigent and to recipients of social assistance. The pacts invariably granted full determination of fees and medical needs to physicians, and simply reimbursed them at a percentage (usually 75 percent) of their fees. Such arrangements became the physicians' preferred method of dealing with government. In this segmented policy regime the role of government was to provide funding assistance so that doctors could provide health care.

Physician-Sponsored Insurance

During the Depression years, the CMA began to develop its own plans for health insurance to capture the concerns and positions of Canada's physicians better than the pending provincial initiatives.

In 1934 the CMA issued a thorough review of the economics of medical practice, which included some comparative studies and set out nineteen principles to guide the development of health insurance.[11] Organized medicine was thus preparing itself for the possibility of national health insurance. A succession of provincial and national medical leaders began to accept the inevitability of a state-sponsored scheme and to concur with a warning voiced as early as 1936: "If we do not socialize ourselves and develop the proper technique of service, Governments will be forced to try their hand" (quoted in Naylor 1986:101).

All this groundwork came to good use when, during the preparations for the 1945 conference, a group of CMA representatives met with the federal government committee in what amounted to an advise-and-consent capacity. The CMA representatives saw to it that the nineteen principles were incorporated into official policy. Government's ready acquiescence was influenced by its traditional deference to the medical profession, interest group power politics aside. Accordingly, the government's draft bill was unanimously endorsed at the next national meeting of the CMA. Canada's organized physicians had become "fully reconciled to, if not enthusiastic about" the inevitability of public health insurance, recognizing it as an important route to expansion and upgrading of the profession (Taylor 1978:132). In addition, physicians clearly preferred the government plans, which they could apparently influence, over the consumer-controlled commercial insurance plans, which were spreading.

At this point in 1944, federalism approached a unique juncture whereby organized medicine and the federal government were poised for mutually supportive roles and relations in health care. Medical consent for a federal initiative that condoned professional prerogatives offered an extraordinary opportunity to national policymakers. That they failed to seize the moment became a major setback. In the debates and political maneuverings on the draft bill, both before and after the 1945 Conference, the positions of the medical profession were subjected to intensive scrutiny. These positions were contradicted by organized labor and farmers' groups, who demanded more "socialization" (lay control of administration and fees, as well as universal and free coverage to avoid a two-tier system). Eventually, organized medicine's unease about its joint venture with government began to intensify. By the time politicians also began to waver and engage in "strategic delay" of health insurance legislation, organized medicine itself was agitating for suspension (Naylor 1986:132). It turned its attention instead to budding physician-sponsored prepayment plans that ensured greater medical control over clinical practice and physicians' incomes. Contestations over the formerly honored separation between medical and governmental spheres and increasing efforts by government actors to become involved in funding arrangements for medical care chipped away at the hold of a segmented policy regime.

Hospital Insurance:
Provincial Initiatives/Federal Support (1948–1958)

The impasse left by the 1945 conference did not last long. Although the conference proposals themselves did not directly shape the next stages of policy development, a new pattern of policy-making began to emerge: The provinces took the initiative in planning and implementation, and future conferences officially sanctioned provincial efforts. By 1950 all the provinces had acted on the understanding that they could negotiate their own tax agreements with the federal government, transferring their jurisdictional prerogatives in return for federal grants. Targeted health grants were introduced in 1948 and initiated research, surveys, and specific programs.[12] The health grants program became, in the prime minister's own words, "the first stages in the development of a comprehensive health insurance plan for all Canadians" (quoted in Taylor 1978:164). Moreover, one of the spinoffs of the grants—annual meetings to review expenditures, creating an opportunity for valuable exchange of information, ideas, and motivation—indirectly reset the dynamics of federalism toward a return to centralized coordination of provincial activities.

The hospital construction grants also encouraged several provinces to undertake the development of hospital insurance. Although each province had its own reason for implementing hospital insurance, in all provinces there was more agreement in this area than on medical insurance.[13] Also, by the 1950s advances in technology and more powerful unionization, among other factors, were precipitating rising hospital costs. Despite the expense, patients (many of whom were inadequately covered by insurance) and third-party payers were demanding more and better hospital care.[14] By the time of the next federal/provincial conference, the situation was ripe for the resumption of a federal government role. A transition in policy regimes began and slowly uprooted the grasp of segmented roles and relations.

Federal Intervention in Provincial Domains

The process of federalism that had been sanctioned by the 1945 conference rested on the principle that the federal government would assist provincial initiatives upon request. The most significant initiative was Saskatchewan's early venture into the domain of hospital insurance.[15] By 1947 Saskatchewan had put into effect a universal, compulsory, hospital insurance system paid through social insurance. The provincial government contributed its portion of payments out of general revenue. Although municipal councils collected the premiums, a centralized commission administered the program. The plan covered all medically necessary hospital services, with extra charges only for accommodations superior to standard ward coverage. As the other provinces considered their options, they learned first from Saskatchewan, and then they revisited the proposals that had been put forward at the 1945 conference.

Three other provinces set up hospital insurance programs, but none were as exemplary as Saskatchewan's. British Columbia's experience with overly complicated administration was a learning tool for other provinces.[16] Alberta also developed a patchwork system of hospital insurance, incrementally adding groups of eligible populations and allowing regions and municipalities to decide their own degree of centralized/decentralized administration. The only other province besides Saskatchewan with a coherent system of hospital insurance in place by the time of the 1955 conference was Newfoundland. Its cottage-hospital system covered nearly half the province's population. But the other provinces eschewed the principles of provincial ownership and salaried physicians that underlay Newfoundland's cottage-hospitals.

Federalism Overtakes the Provinces—By Design

Canadian-style federalism is based on cooperation and majority rule. For it to function well, one of the two largest provinces must be a willing partner. In most cases Ontario has played a critical role in the success of federalism. Given its flourishing private insurance industry, it is surprising and significant that Ontario was a decisive actor in the introduction of hospital insurance in Canada. The insurance industry's failure to provide consistent and fair coverage was one reason. The premier himself, Leslie Frost, had been a victim of self-serving insurance practices; to his dismay his health policy was canceled when he turned 60. He also sensed that public health insurance was inevitable and that the only question was one of timing.[17]

At an upcoming federal/provincial conference scheduled for 1955, the Liberal prime minister wanted to discuss only intergovernmental fiscal arrangements and unemployment insurance. Ontario's Conservative premier insisted that health insurance be on the agenda as well. The 1955 conference did not come to any agreement on health insurance, but ended with the appointment of a joint federal/provincial committee to study the issue. The committee sessions went beyond information exchange to actual negotiations between the provincial and federal representatives (all ministers of health and finance). By January 1956 they ended with a statement on the federal role in assisting the provinces in the development of hospital insurance. The main items were the following: The federal government would begin assistance as soon as a majority of the provinces representing a majority of the Canadian people agreed to proceed with hospital insurance plans; priority would be given to diagnostic services and in-patient hospital care; the federal contribution would pertain to normal operating and maintenance costs and not capital or administrative costs; the federal contribution would be 25 percent of the average per capita costs for hospital services in Canada as a whole and 25 percent of the average per capita costs in the province itself, multiplied by the number of insured people in the province. It was up to the provinces to accept this position. The ball had been put back on the provincial side, and Ontario accepted it.

Provincial Implementation

Ontario provided a test for one of the chief contingencies in federalism—where and how action is to be initiated. Both the 1945 and 1955 conferences had left certain features of federal/provincial roles and relations unclear. Would the federal government lead the provinces and provide facilitative funding to each province ready and willing to begin the process of change? Would the provinces take the initiative using their own mechanisms to establish their own programs and then get federal funding to continue what they were already doing on their own, in which case, could they decide themselves when and even if they wanted federal assistance and its accompanying interference? Or would both central and decentralized actors exercise mutually supportive and more flexible rights and responsibilities? These contingencies were never fully resolved. They were determined by the particular configurations of power prevailing in particular circumstances.

By 1957 only three provinces had accepted the federal terms; British Columbia, Alberta, and Saskatchewan already had hospital plans operating and were eager to accept federal assistance. After further study and hearings in Ontario, the premier was prepared to begin hospital insurance. But he did not want to wait for two more provinces to come on board before receiving federal start-up assistance. An exchange of letters between the prime minister and the premier ended in capitulation by the federal government.[18] With a signed agreement between Ontario and Ottawa, a bill was introduced in the House of Commons, and after the usual debate, the Hospital and Diagnostic Services Act (HIDS) passed unanimously in 1957. During these long negotiations, Manitoba had adopted its own plan, eventually making Ontario the fifth province in which action was pending. Within days of the passage of HIDS, Prince Edward Island became the sixth province to sign on, making moot the new prime minister's announcement of his intention to cancel the "sixth province" requirement. By 1961 all ten provinces had joined the federal hospital insurance system.

National legislation changed above all how hospital care was financed. Individuals no longer paid premiums to commercial insurance companies; instead, they paid, in most cases through payroll deductions, a similar amount for the provincial government premium that provided a standard insurance "policy." Hospitals no longer charged individuals or insurance companies; they charged the provincial government instead, and the certainty of reimbursement improved revenues for some hospitals. Hospitals continued to be governed by their same boards of trustees—private individuals for the most part, although provincial governments acquired the right to appoint public trustees (Evans 1984:183). Where applicable and possible, insurance companies' structures and/or personnel were transformed or absorbed into the provincial hospital commission. In all provinces the role of commercial insurance in hospital care shifted to one of coverage for "extras" not included in the government plan, such as private beds. In some provinces commercial carriers continued as before to administer medical insurance (for physician services), although without the hospital care component. The initial transition to hospital insurance had been relatively painless.[19]

The HIDS Act introduced a new order in hospital/government relations. It is possible but not altogether accurate to say that passage of the HIDS legislation represents a reverse form of federalism in Canada, one in which the provinces assumed leadership over the federal government. It is more accurate to indicate that the HIDS Act and the subsequent measures that fleshed out its terms bestowed onto the federal government an unprecedented degree of command over what provinces and hospitals were to do, thereby establishing an interventionist policy regime. The federal government required uniform terms and standards across the country. The basic conditions that had to be fulfilled for participation were simple enough and easily met: Each hospital had to provide specified minimum services; each province had to offer comprehensive, universal, and free coverage (although small premiums or copayments were permissible); and each province's plan had to be portable (that is, residents moving or visiting from another province had to be covered). To enable the poorer provinces to meet these requirements, the federal government tightened its power of equalization (which refers to a funding formula under which the federal contribution is less to the better-endowed provinces and more to the poorer ones). Hospital governing boards remained independent but exercised their prerogatives within fiscal constraints.[20] Provincial governments were affected by the HIDS legislation in a new way, for it marked the first time they had to comply with such detailed requirements in any policy field. Besides issuing new regulations, the federal government also acquired oversight powers to audit costs that were shared, which also meant more provincial government oversight of each hospital's budget (Glaser 1980:II-9). In the same way that the federal level of government acquired greater control over hospital care vis-à-vis the provinces, provincial ministries of health acquired greater control over hospital budgets vis-à-vis the boards of governance.

Thus, an interventionist policy regime emerged, although gently at first. HIDS was a major piece of national legislation that concentrated at the federal level more political power in health care than ever before. Private insurance companies experienced this intervention more sharply than any other set of health care actors. The moderate and supportive nature of federal government intervention (especially when compared to the more intrusive cases of Britain and the United States) set a concomitant spirit of cooperation between the provinces and the federal government in determining, for instance, when provinces would enter the national program. Canada is unique among the three countries for its early capacity to accept accommodation when necessary. The practical knowledge would come in handy later, when tensions worsened.

Profession and Government: Preparing for Change

The medical profession's support of the hospital insurance plan was mixed at best.[21] In the main, however, physicians were resigned to hospital insurance and recognized that it was probably a first step toward broader health insurance, but the details of the bigger picture remained unclear. Accordingly, as the bandwagon of hospital insurance rolled on, the profession geared up to adopt a role in shaping the next step: medical insurance. The CMA began by insisting that hospital insurance be separated from reimbursement of physicians, whether medical care was provided within or outside the hospital. It sharpened its position by stating that all physicians should be paid on a fee-for-service basis.[22] Its political activities began to lay the groundwork for a vivid division in the interests of the medical profession as opposed to government actors.

Medical Care Insurance: Governmental Prodding/ Professional Acquiescence (1958–1968)

The passage of the HIDS Act created the "other shoe" syndrome, as Taylor (1978:352) aptly puts it. Several provinces had already begun to confront the issue of physician-reimbursement insurance after World War II, and the HIDS Act seemed to offer an encouraging climate for them to continue. But the forays were fraught with increasing tensions over autonomous rights and responsibilities in health care. It is appropriate to begin this section with the position of the medical profession.

Government Intervention in Professional Domains

Insofar as the medical profession in Canada supported the principle of a public program as early as 1944, we might say that it has never been as consistently or adamantly opposed to national health insurance as its counterpart in the United States. In addition to their acceptance of government endeavors, several provincial medical associations experimented with various prepayment plans. Physicians in the western provinces united with consumer organizations in the spirit of the cooperative movement that marked the 1930s. In the 1940s and later, several provincial medical associations started their own profession-sponsored prepaid health insurance plans.[23]

After the 1945 federal/provincial conference, the CMA turned its attention to these provincial ventures, and in 1949 it officially changed its policy to one of support for voluntary prepaid insurance. It specifically opposed a government scheme but continued to support government subsidy of the needy within a voluntary prepaid plan. By 1951 the CMA had formalized a "federal" relationship among the provincial physician-sponsored programs with the creation of Trans-Canada Medical Services. (Its name later changed to Trans-Canada Medical Plans [TCMP].) In the professional activism that followed, which included the CMA negotiating TCMP contracts with several large employers, the CMA was enacting a strategy of promoting and solidifying the profession-sponsored plans so that if and when calls for national health insurance came about, they would necessarily be framed by ongoing physician-controlled developments. As it set about its endeavors, the profession began to justify ever more concretely the necessity of medical control over health care administration so as to ensure medical autonomy in the dispensation of knowledge. The "federal" relationship between the profession and the government became entrenched in its historical roots in a segmented policy regime: Each set of actors posed its power as preemptory to the assertions of the other. And with the government hesitant to impose its will, the principle of mutually exclusive domains reigned.

Professional Opposition

By the late 1950s organized medicine had to swallow a heavy dose of reality and was forced to change its tactics to bolster its strategy. The growth of commercial insurance made the private sector a formidable contender for domination in the process of constructing a framework for medical (that is, physician) care policy. The CMA had become critical of the inadequacies and inconsistencies of commercial plans, and advocated its own profession-sponsored form of prepayment as a more "all-inclusive, efficient, and sound" system of medical insurance (quoted in Taylor 1978:28). However, soon after the creation of the TCMP, it was becoming clear that the differences among the provincial association plans could not be easily harmonized to compete effectively against commercial insurance companies.[24] The CMA, recognizing the benefits to be reaped from repeating the tactic of collaboration with one opponent against an enemy common to both, sent a delegation to the 1960 Canadian Health Insurance Association (CHIA) conference to discuss issues of mutual interest. The conference members agreed to unite their efforts and to construct a broader base of support for their nongovernmental approach to medical-care insurance.[25]

Certain of the rational appeal of their mission and hoping to forestall pending action on health insurance by the government in Saskatchewan, the 1960 conference requested, among other things, that the prime minister, Progressive Conservative John Diefenbaker, establish a commission of inquiry on health insurance. Officially, the CMA called for "removing the consideration of health and health insurance from the hectic arena of political controversy" (quoted in Naylor 1986:191). But in stating that the mandate of the commission should be "assessing the health needs and resources of Canada with a view to recommending methods of ensuring the highest standard of health care for all Canadians," it was clearly expecting to shape discussion of the issue (quoted in Naylor 1986:191). The Royal Commission on Health Services (the Hall Commission) issued its report in 1964. To everyone's astonishment the commission rejected completely any alternatives to public insurance and proposed a system parallel to the hospital insurance model. It insisted on uniform terms and conditions of coverage, which could not be achieved through voluntary and commercial plans. The commission's own survey had found that these plans were not as widespread as their representatives had claimed; only one-half of the population was covered for medical care, and inadequately at that. Its main concessions to the medical profession's position were to recognize freedom of choice both for patients and for "free and self-governing professionals," and to endorse fee-for-service as the most practicable method of reimbursement for Canada (quoted in Taylor 1978:346). Acting as an arm of government, the Royal Commission extended the scope of a budding interventionist policy regime to include medical care.

Within days of the release of the Hall Report, the CMA held its annual national conference, at which its independent position was reiterated and its resolve strengthened. The medical profession in Canada had by now become a visible and vocal presence in the health policy debate. However, the task of influencing that debate was becoming more formidable as support for medical care insurance steadily mounted on the part of both provincial governments and the public at large.[26] Moreover, the turn of events in Saskatchewan was becoming a foreboding test case for the future of medical-care insurance.

Professional/Provincial Developments

The confrontation over medical care in Saskatchewan was particularly dramatic evidence of the strain that had become lodged in professional/governmental relations. Saskatchewan's early establishment of municipal doctor systems and supportive environment for voluntary prepayment plans had epitomized smooth relations between professional and governmental actors. By the time hospital insurance became public policy, with Saskatchewan leading the way, the province had developed a variety of methods for paying physicians. It seemed to be the ideal location for sowing the seeds of medical care insurance. The funding that became available with the implementation of the HIDS Act was interpreted by Saskatchewan's provincial government leaders as available for the extension of medical-care insurance, and so the question arose as to which alternative should become the basis of a provincial plan. Eventually the debate focused on two models: compulsory, universal public insurance reimbursing physicians on a salary or per capita basis; or voluntary, physician-controlled, fee-for-service plans. The increasingly confrontational positions of the provincial government and the Saskatchewan College of Physicians and Surgeons (which was combined with the provincial medical association) came to a head in 1959, when the government presented to the provincial parliament its draft bill for a compulsory, universal medical insurance plan. Months of debate and acrimony ensued, climaxed by an unprecedented, bitter strike by Saskatchewan's physicians.[27] The agreement that was finally signed in 1962 was hard-won and tenuous, each side dissatisfied with its concessions.[28]

The tensions in Saskatchewan precipitated preventive action in other provinces, especially those that preferred less "socialist" routes than Saskatchewan had followed, despite a groundswell in favor of medical-care insurance. Governments in British Columbia, Alberta, and Ontario all backed the voluntary plans of their (and the national) medical associations.[29] In addition, commercial insurance for the nonindigent also flourished in Alberta and Ontario.[30] Thus, by the time the Hall Report was issued the CMA and the CHIA had found ready allies in those provinces wishing to minimize the role of the federal government in health insurance. But this base of support was fragile, because provincial governments were at the same time using their relations with the medical associations to foil upcoming confrontations with the federal government over constitutional issues.

The 1964 release of the Hall Report on medical-care insurance found the medical profession in a vulnerable position, in its internal as well as its external relations. The profession had lost the battle in Saskatchewan doubly—suffering defeat both on the plan itself and in its propitious consequences for physician incomes.[31] Most important, the profession's support for its own physician-sponsored plans began to wane as these became less physician- and more consumer-oriented.[32] With the TCMP plans no longer serving physician interests, the CMA voted in 1964 to endorse the multiple-carrier concept as its preferred method of insuring the population. Organized medicine had been reduced to clinging to fee-for-service with extra-billing privileges as the core feature of its autonomy. Ironically, the only shelter it could find was through the agencies of multiple carriers that were controlled more by consumer and market interests than by those of physicians.

By 1964 the profession's internal divisions were weakening its positions. The CMA's rank and file had undergone a generational change, with older supporters of government-subsidized health care contending with a younger, more militant group whose rising incomes made them more protective of their interests and adverse to any third-party interference in direct patient billing (Naylor 1986:228). Although the latter group was in a minority, its voice was loud and its position was clear: Any government plan would necessarily need ample provision for physicians to opt out. The

CMA had already invoked the principle of provincial rights to bolster its opposition to a government plan; the only argument remaining was that surely government would not impose a plan that did not have the profession's cooperation and support. Its flailing efforts revealed that its overall leverage had faded. It could only respond with relief to the concessions the federal government offered: Opting out and extra billing (as long as it was not excessive) would both be allowed in the new proposals, even though both had been opposed in the Hall Report. The medical profession's continued engagement in negotiating concessions also meant that it would accept the upcoming legislation (known now as Medicare), albeit reluctantly, on behalf of those of its members who were willing to participate. Yet it also continued to voice the opposition of those who chose to exit. The stance of the medical profession had created strong oppositional forces in the relations of federalism, which meant that the other side (in this case, government in general, both provincial and federal) either would have to be very forceful in imposing its position or would have to retreat for the sake of harmony. The resolution came from the particular circumstances of federalism extant at the time. It reinforced the parameters of an interventionist policy regime, but it also reminded all actors of prior autonomous rights and responsibilities.

Expanding Federal Intervention in Provincial Domains

The Hall Report was as momentous for its consequences on provincial/federal as on professional/governmental relations. By the time the report was issued in 1964, not only were some provinces formulating their official support for voluntary insurance plans, but several, most notably Ontario and Quebec, were becoming seriously opposed to the shared-cost principle that had grounded the fiscal terms of the relationship between the provincial and federal governments. Under the HIDS Act, the use of conditional grants-in-aid to establish national standards had included a strong federal role in licensing and inspecting hospitals. Although the outcomes had been positive in terms of hospital standards, provincial actors were aware of being manipulated. Moreover, events in Quebec had shifted back toward a reassertion of provincial prerogatives.[33] With their indignation at federal interference growing and their own bureaucracies expanding, provincial governments were feeling both more self-sufficient and more powerful. Their centrifugal vision of federalism was acquiring greater intensity.

The Hall Report diverted this impulse. It stipulated that universal coverage and uniform terms and conditions of coverage within each province be the criteria of provincial qualification for federal funding. It claimed that only a compulsory system could hope to overcome the provincial disparities in health care and insurance coverage. And it called for federal/provincial agreements similar to those undertaken to implement HIDS. The report upheld the grant method of financing, asserting that Canada "could have a tax-financed health service, run by the provinces with federal grants-in-aid based on fiscal need" (quoted in Mahler 1987:92). It seemed, in other words, to envision centripetal forces driving the machinery of federalism. The clear duality that had emerged between provincial government and medical association preferences, on the one hand, and federal preferences, on the other, meant that the time was ripe for compromise to avoid a stalemate and, more important, to preserve the federal system.

When the Hall Report was issued, a new Liberal government was in power, with a new prime minister, Lester Pearson. The years out of office had strengthened the party's resolve to live up to its pledge, first made in 1919, to enact national health insurance. At the same time, its return to office had been beset by fallen political fortunes and much political in-fighting. In the compromises that followed the Hall Report, the federal government seemed once again to capitulate to the provinces. But this turned out to be only a short-term view. Intensive discussions to work out realistic options for funding arrangements, administrative structures, and a clear understanding of rights and responsibilities preceded the federal government's presentation of its proposals at the 1965 federal/provincial conference. The many conditions that had permeated the hospital insurance proposals were simplified now to four criteria for provincial participation in national medical-care insurance: Provincial programs had to be comprehensive, covering all the services provided by general practitioners and specialists; the plans had to be universal, covering all residents in a province on uniform terms and conditions; the programs had to be administered by a public agency; and benefits had to be transportable to residents moving to another province or temporarily absent from the province. Unlike under HIDS, no federal audits of provincial plans were necessary. And to complement these loose features of the new federal relationship in medical-care insurance, a simplified funding formula was proposed, whereby the federal government would contribute the same amount to each province: one-half of the national per capita cost of the insurance system. Finally, the federal government offered to establish a Health Resources Fund for medical training to round out its contributions. The role of the federal government was thus transformed from confrontational to facilitative. And in its assistance, the federal government had clearly acquired more than a secondary role in the provision of health care. Without compromising their goals, federal government actors pragmatically devised decentralized methods of implementation.[34] They conceded on the means, not the ends. The result remained the establishment of an interventionist policy regime, but its tone of intrusiveness was mitigated by cooperation.

The Medical Care Insurance (Medicare) bill was introduced in Parliament in 1965, debated for months, and underwent one final federal concession: delay in its implementation until one year after Canada's 1967 centennial celebration. But pass it did, with only two dissenting votes. The bill contained no requirement for a minimum number of participating provinces. When Medicare was first enacted, only two provinces (Saskatchewan and British Columbia) qualified. Within two-and-one-half years all were participants. The transition to full national health insurance was difficult for most provinces: Quebec suffered a bruising strike by its physicians; Alberta and Ontario eventually had to phase out most of their voluntary insurance carriers; and the Maritime provinces continually suffered funding shortages and administrative inadequacies. Nevertheless, the achievement of public insurance for medical care was a watershed in Canadian federalism. It demonstrated the possibility of a coherent national framework within which provincial variations in capacity and choice were allowed full play. An unprecedented measure of federal intervention had been necessary to attain the legislation, but once it was in place, roles and relations returned to a modus vivendi of respect for traditional rights and responsibilities without, however, retreating to the framework of separate domains. In fact, a tone of accommodation rather than forbearance was introduced in the sociopolitical relations of health care. This coexistence of different policy regime norms was short-lived, however. As cost concerns grew in the next phase, tensions and contradictions erupted.

The Struggle for Control Over the System
(1971–1984)

The compromises necessary to pass the hospital and medical-care insurance systems soon enough led to problems and dissatisfactions as the costs of health care burgeoned. Interpretation of "the problem" differed, of course, among the main sets of actors. The federal government found that its open-ended contribution to health care costs was growing at an unprecedented and uncontrollable rate and that this was due only in small part to inflation.[35] Shared-cost funding had enabled the federal government to shape provincial priorities in the programs and create national program standards, but control of overall expenditure was more ephemeral. For built into the funding arrangements was an incentive for provinces to spend only on insured items, since they were contributing in effect only half of the costs,[36] and to retreat from experimenting with other, perhaps less expensive, forms of health care, because these were not cost-shared. Since hospital care was first to be insured, and its use accelerated by construction grants, its costs, already the highest in health care, rose inexorably.

For their part, provincial governments were becoming increasingly resentful of federal interference, especially in the oversights and audits developed to assure compliance with conditions for receipt of Medicare funds. They also felt increasingly constrained in their ability to control costs because of federal regulations pertaining to HIDS.[37] The differences among the provinces became more intense as their demands for federal withdrawal increased. The richer provinces, annoyed with the strings attached and with watching their tax credits siphoned to the poorer provinces, wanted to reduce federal funding to its minimum. The poorer provinces, concerned because the cost-sharing formula extended more funding to provinces with higher costs and expenditures, wanted more federal funds directed to them. All provinces were united, however, in wanting more autonomy in determining their own program and spending priorities.

Ironically, physicians were the only actors who tolerated the health insurance system in its early stages, because the bitter pill they had to swallow with the passage of Medicare was sweetened by the extra-billing privileges from which they were reaping enormous benefits. Both physician incomes and the number of physicians increased considerably in the years following enactment of Medicare. The Medicare legislation also included provisions for expanding education, training, and research. Nevertheless, physicians eventually found grounds to complain that the health care system as a whole was becoming dangerously underfunded. All around it became clear that the funding arrangements of health insurance had to be rethought. It was also clear, however, that funding alone, not Medicare itself, would be subject to negotiation, for the public popularity of the program made its retraction or retrenchment politically unthinkable. Negotiations on a new funding system began in 1971. Its first stage, which affected primarily provincial/federal relations, took six years to settle; its second stage, pertaining primarily to physicians, took another seven years to legislate and has still not been completely settled. Federal government actors began to sharpen their tools of intervention but refrained from using them too forcefully.

Wavering Federal Intervention

When in the 1970s the pendulum of federalism swung back to the provinces, the politics of taxation provided the mechanism for change. The constitution allows only the federal government to collect personal and corporate income taxes; it does so on behalf of the provinces as well as itself and reimburses the provincial share through tax transfers. In the discussions and negotiations on funding arrangements following the enactment of Medicare, all parties turned to tax transfers as a mechanism to reduce federal grant-giving and the provincial dependence and federal power it had created. By increasing the provinces' tax credits (or increasing their tax "room," as it is called), the provinces would have as much funding as before, approximating their population size as before, but there would be no need for federal conditions. The arrangements that were concluded reaffirmed the continuing necessity of a special equalization formula to compensate for the disparities in provincial income levels, but beyond this main federal role, a return to provincial control of funding for health care was envisioned.

Respecifying Funding Responsibilities

By the early 1970s representatives of all levels of government agreed that the 50–50 cost-sharing arrangement should be replaced by a tax shift.[38] The federal government vacated a fixed percentage of tax points (12 personal and 1 corporate income tax points) as additional tax room for the provinces, to be used for three social programs (hospital care, medical care, and education) with no strings attached. The federal government also extended a per capita block grant for each of the three programs, amounting to about one-half of the previous federal contribution and requiring only that the same four basic principles instituted for Medicare (comprehensive services, universality, portability, public administration) be met as before—but now, in the spirit of a reduced federal role, without detailed auditing to confirm compliance. An additional per capita payment was included to be used for extended or noninstitutional health care services, such as nursing home care, other intermediate care, home care, and ambulatory services.[39] This was the only feature of the new agreement specifically related to the substance of health care. Finally, a one-time transitional adjustment payment compensated the provinces for their reorganization costs. The package of changes was assembled as the 1977 Federal/Provincial Fiscal Arrangements and Established Programs Financing Act (EPFA). It had taken five years of fiscal testing and negotiations to construct a new form of "fiscal federalism," as this relationship came to be called. But because the terms of the arrangement were confined to funding alone and were not complemented by a reconstruction of the politics, provision, and delivery of health care, its success was circumscribed.

Retreats in Federalism

The consequences of the legislation partially fulfilled its purposes. The federal government was relieved of unpredictable and unstable health care expenditures, in return for which it relinquished considerable leverage in shaping national standards (Taylor 1986:16). The provinces gained greater discretion over spending priorities, but with this power came the burden of decisions about cost control. The provinces turned first to the horrendous task of cutting hospital costs. Targeted measures were attempted. But hospital closures proved to be politically difficult to carry out, and converting hospital facilities and units to nonacute and outpatient care was physically difficult (Van Loon 1978:467). Moreover, the consequences of increased labor action among unionized hospital workers was proving costly. Thus, the apparent swing in the pendulum of federalism back to the provinces found the provinces unprepared and incapable of fully exercising their newfound power. Although decentralization had seemed imminent, its administrative foundation was weak.

Because of the floundering that followed, the EPFA was criticized as offering too little too late. The transfer of power it promised was more abstract than real; it carried no assistance, whether administrative, financial, or conceptual, for the provinces to redirect their health care spending. Both hospital payment and fee-for-service reimbursement, the two most costly features in health care, seemed impervious to provincial government tinkering. And, as had happened in an earlier era of shifting federal/provincial relations, the federal government seemed to withdraw "from active engagement in the direction and development of Canada's health care services" (Mendelson and Sullivan 1990:11). To the extent that this assessment held, it was temporary. With the benefit of hindsight, it can be argued that the federal government had not withdrawn. Instead, its role was changing from concretely facilitating the provinces in their efforts to conform to federal guidelines to handling potentially destabilizing consequences of provincial attempts to establish provincially based rules for universal and equitable health care provision. The EPFA gave the provinces the incentive to try to control costs on their own. Their responses introduced mechanisms that became more effective with time.[40]

Intervention Returns

Nevertheless, within a few years of its implementation, the EPFA had created considerable political turmoil. The apparent withdrawal of the federal government, caused by its loss of oversight powers under the EPFA legislation, together with fumbling efforts to control costs on the part of provincial governments and the diffusion of accountability that resulted, created another void waiting to be filled. With health care costs continuing to grow, all parties were suspected of not living up to their responsibilities in health care. A conference of provincial health care ministers asked the newly elected Conservative federal government to summon a commission of inquiry and agreed that it be headed by the same former Supreme Court justice, Emmet Hall, responsible for the 1964 Hall Report. The Health Services Review Committee, reporting in 1980, delivered the first thorough review of the national health insurance program. The committee found that provincial governments were not diverting funds from health care, as had been alleged, but added that some provinces were endangering the principle of reasonable access by charging premiums and user fees.[41] It recommended that all provinces use tax-based methods to finance their programs and that user fees be eliminated.

The next Liberal government seized the opportunity offered by growing criticisms of Medicare to establish a parliamentary investigation into the whole question of fiscal federalism and its various policy components. This all-party House of Commons task force decided that "the proper role for the federal government is the formulation, monitoring and enforcement of conditions on its financial support of provincial programs."[42] It recommended that the hospital insurance and medical care acts be consolidated; that clear program conditions be established, along with explicit criteria constituting noncompliance; that federal financing be withheld to vagrant provinces; and that the recommendations of the Hall Commission be adopted.[43] The task force explicitly rejected organized medicine's argument that the health care system was underfunded. It also commented on the expansion of expenditures in health care, noting that the only necessary area of expansion was in preventive health care; medical and hospital services, on the other hand, had been wastefully overemphasized. This recommendation, together with the federal government's determination to cancel the Revenue Guarantee tax transfers, eventually led to a cap on increases in government spending on statutory social programs. The task force, in effect, folded the process of fiscal federalism into the more important collective need for federal leadership in setting national program standards. A committee of inquiry once again became a mechanism not only for reinserting the federal government into health care, but also for specifying a new federal role in health care. I elaborate its dimensions later.

Profession and Government: Consolidating Intervention

Doctors' billing practices and payments changed little when Medicare was first enacted. Those changes that did occur were improvements, simplifying billing procedures by establishing a single payer, and regularizing and increasing payments. Most provincial governments adopted without alteration the existing schedule of benefits used by physicians and reimbursed them fully, or nearly so, for their services. The Medicare Act allowed each province to negotiate the parameters of a fee schedule with its representative medical association. Most provinces continue to follow a standard procedure: Negotiations, conducted either annually or every two or three years, first yield a rate of increase in the total amount of reimbursement; provincial governments then leave it to the medical profession to decide how to distribute fee changes among specialties and procedures. Each provincial medical association conducts its own internal negotiations to settle this matter. There is no government interference in the proceedings within the profession. Lastly, the provincial government adopts the association's specific schedule of fees for individual procedures as the basis of its reimbursement.

It was fully understood when Medicare was first enacted that some difference between charges/fees and reimbursement might occur; such differences are a fact of life in all third-party plans.[44] Physicians' estimates of their actual costs are particularly likely to exceed government's budgetary limitations. The Medicare legislation allowed for a practice called extra billing or balance billing, whereby doctors could charge patients directly for the difference between their own rates and the provincial reimbursement they received.[45] Doctors who engaged in extra billing were said to opt out of Medicare. They were required to inform their patients of their billing practices before providing their services. Most opted-out doctors refrained from extra billing the elderly and needy.[46]

Over time, the disparity between the profession's fee schedules and the provinces' actual reimbursements grew. By the 1970s the physician payment portion of provincial health budgets had grown at a faster rate than hospital expenditures. Provincial governments had little control over clinical practice and the physician-controlled standards governing the content of care and its manner of delivery, whether in private practices or in hospitals. Weak provincial control was exacerbated by a generalized governmental concession to reimburse those services deemed by physicians to be "medically necessary."[47] Certain provinces attempted to monitor physicians' billing practices, but unsuccessfully for the most part.[48] Most provinces responded to rising expenditures by restricting the annual increases in physician fee schedules. But their success in controlling physician billings was limited; from 1972 to

1984 the provinces cut fees by 18 percent in real terms while total billing claims rose by 17 percent (Terris 1990:31). Nevertheless, during this same period the real value of medical fees fell by 15.9 percent (Wahn 1992:723);[49] that is, physicians were providing more services to maintain their incomes, but they were not increasing their incomes. Provinces had become ever more cost conscious after the implementation of the 1977 EPFA arrangements and began in earnest to engage in cost control measures, but no one was satisfied with the results.

The working relationship between the medical profession and government visibly deteriorated when national wage and price controls were imposed in 1975. Although physicians were allotted some annual increases in their reimbursements, they tried to recoup their losses when the freeze was lifted in 1978, by demanding extra-large increases, as much as 44 percent in British Columbia.[50] In addition, after the controls a number of physicians chose to opt out of the provincial plans, increasing the number of physicians who were extra-billing. Over and above using extra billing as a safety valve for maintaining their incomes, the medical profession in Canada seized on the practice as the last vestige of autonomy in the face of encroaching government interference. Provincial governments responded by squeezing the rate of increase in annual allotments for physician payments, offering much less than the profession requested. As a result, the discrepancy between physicians' rates and provincial reimbursements became markedly out of line. The greatest difference was in Ontario, where physicians claimed that the schedule used by the provincial government for reimbursement was 25 percent lower than the one calculated by the Ontario Medical Association (OMA) to reflect physicians' total costs. As extra billing and the additional user fees being charged in some provinces for hospitalization grew across the country, the federal government became alarmed that these practices were contradicting the stated purpose of the national legislation: to provide reasonable access to health care.[51]

When the 1980 Hall Report, which had attested to financial abuse, and the 1981 Parliamentary Task Force Report were issued, the Liberals were back in power. Minister of Health Monique Bégin, who was committed to following through on the recommendations of the reports, tried first the strategy of "moral suasion" to forge voluntary measures for controlling extra billing and

user fees.[52] When this failed to produce adequate results, she commissioned a public opinion poll. Buoyed by the overwhelming
response against extra billing, the Liberal government decided to
take the legislative route. After debates and several revisions, a
draft bill was presented to Parliament. It proposed amendments to
HIDS and Medicare that consolidated them, reinforced their four
basic conditions (comprehensive, universal, portable, and publicly
administered provision) with additional clarification and redefinition, and added a fifth condition: accessibility.[53] The bill became
the Canada Health Act (CHA). Parliament passed it unanimously in
April 1984; however, political contention surrounded government/
professional relations, as we will see. Passage of the CHA represents
an unprecedented assertion of federal government authority in the
field of health care. It is also the pinnacle event in the rule of an
interventionist policy regime in Canada.

Tightening Federal Control:
A Continuing Struggle (1984–)

Up to this point the discussion of health policy development in
Canada has focused on the macrorelations of federalism. Constitutional inconsistencies and obscurities prompted government
actors to clarify jurisdictional disputes and determine financial
responsibilities more appropriately. Federalism resembled a pendulum of shifting power and control in the politics of social policy.
Health care itself has seemed to be almost secondary to the question of who has final authority in deciding how much each party
should pay. The passage of the Canada Health Act represents a
unique milestone for settling issues of governance, and in so doing
it facilitated a shift in the terms of the debate toward concerns
about health care itself. Prior to the CHA, the federal government
had not directly addressed microlevel issues of provision and delivery of health care, leaving these to provinces, hospital boards, and
medical associations to work out. The federal government adopted
the challenge posed by the CHA and began to test its broader capacities to be involved in such issues as what kind of care is best for
whom and what constitutes right- and wrong-doing in health care.
    Because the provinces and the medical profession responded pos-
itively to these wide-ranging discussions about health care, a new
form of federalism has begun to emerge. Its features are still un-

clear. It includes the main actors involved thus far, but as discussed in Chapter 5, it extends the social relations of health care to the private sector. As the Canada Health Act has settled in, it has steered policy-making toward the principles and norms of an integrative regime. Intermittently, a segmented policy regime, which remains strong in Canada, reappears to assert traditional domains. And occasionally, reversion to an interventionist policy regime occurs to offset centrifugal forces.

Integrative Intergovernmental Activities

The fiscal changes that occurred in the 1970s granted the provinces more control in financing their own health care systems, and in setting and implementing their own priorities in health care. In one main sense this control can be thought of as more symbolic than real: The provinces have not been able actually to cut health care expenditures. When first granted fiscal authority, they had neither the power nor the political will to curtail spending, since Medicare had become an immensely popular program. And with the passage of the Canada Health Act they no longer had the right to jeopardize the achievement of national guidelines.

The CHA required only two specific actions on the part of provinces—to ban user fees for hospital care and to legislate bans on extra billing. (The case of extra billing is elaborated below under professional/governmental relations.) The ban on user fees was neither controversial nor difficult to institute, but the implications for containing hospital costs were profound. Several provinces had levied various forms of user fees at the outset of the hospital insurance system, in order to generate extra revenue and control demand. By the 1980s, for reasons pertaining to both health care and cost control, several provinces had begun to experiment with alternative, noninstitutional forms of delivery. The increasingly pressing need to contain costs reemphasized what had been only slowly dawning since EPFA: that HIDS and Medicare had locked in the hospital as a basis of the health care system and that more concerted effort would be needed to deinstitutionalize the system. Developments toward alternative forms of care have been slow and incremental, which is typical of Canada, but they demonstrate the provinces' earnest concern about unnecessary reliance on expensive hospital care. The following discussion indicates that a great deal of experimentation is under way, in which an unusual flexibility in roles and relations is emerging. It is of interest to note that worries about finances still pertain, but their resolution is being framed more directly than ever before by concerns about health care per se.

1. All provinces are undertaking hospital deinstitutionalization. Following reports at both the provincial and federal levels of government on the inefficiencies and overuse of traditional hospital care, provincial governments tried to cut hospital beds throughout the 1970s. The EPFA offered new tools and renewed motivation. But for the most part, these efforts either failed or produced minimal results.[54] With the Canada Health Act in place, the framework for reducing hospital use broadened to include legislative assistance from the federal government. Deinstitutionalization is in its infancy, but it is at the center of policy discussions. The case of Ontario is illustrative of new directions. Although reductions in the proportion of hospital expenditures within Ontario's health budget are still small,[55] they represent not only top-down enforcement of decisions to contain increases in hospital expenditures, but more important, bottom-up decisions on implementing alternative methods of health care delivery. The provincial government has met with all relevant actors in Ontario's health care system to plan a shift to more outpatient care. The effort is having some success, gradually resulting in both declining acute-care patient-days and reduced annual growth in the operating budgets of hospitals.

In other parts of Canada deinstitutionalization has brought about some novel experiments in transforming hospitals. For example, in New Brunswick different sizes and types of hospitals are sharing services and developing new programs (day surgery and visiting specialty clinics) in an experiment called hospitals without walls (Brown and Ritchie 1992). In British Columbia, the Hospital Innovation Incentive Fund offers a revolving "seed" fund of interest-free loans for efficiency programs (Haazen 1992:81). These and related developments are occurring under the umbrella of the CHA, which allows the federal government to assist the provinces legislatively according to individually negotiated terms while maintaining national standards. Provincial governments have become bolder in undertaking the politically difficult task of deinstitutionalization, knowing they will be backed up by the federal government.

2. Greater use of noninstitutional care (intermediary and community) facilities and programs is the flip side of the deinstitutionalization of hospitals, but it does not occur without considerable diversion of start-up resources.[56] British Columbia has introduced a hospital/community partnership program to enable community-based centers (that is, smaller facilities) to perform certain of the functions formerly housed in hospitals, including disease prevention and health promotion (Haazen 1992:80). The extent to which provinces have been able to expand their noninstitutional care programs for the elderly, who occupy a large proportion of hospital beds, represents not only a planning approach to the utilization of health care resources, but also an appreciation of the role of various social groups in meeting health care needs. In these new endeavors macroplanning has become less interventionist and more oriented toward meshing governmental priorities with local concerns.

3. The longest haul in rational control of resources is in the area of technology acquisition. This is an area in which an interventionist policy regime still appears to rule. The operating and capital budgets of hospitals remain strictly separated in most provinces, so that provincial governments can control purchases. New technology is acquired through special requests that are carefully reviewed by provincial ministries. When this route fails, hospitals must turn to savings in global budgeting or special fund-raising efforts.[57] Existing technology is maintained through depreciation allowances. Some provinces, such as British Columbia, have introduced more systematic projections of technological needs based on population/demographic variables (Haazen 1992). Ontario has taken a micromanagement approach to the acquisition of computerized tomography scanners only, identifying hospital and population criteria for purchase approval, but the policy has been weakly enforced.[58] All in all, global budgeting has achieved some control over use of hospital resources. It functions as the outer framework of expenditure decisions within which hospital personnel (above all, physicians) determine eligibility and engage in implicit rationing through queuing. Technically speaking, this pattern could be said to represent a coordinated effort to contain costs, but because the outcome ultimately restricts the level of health care offered to many patients, it has raised considerable controversy.

4. There has been significant encouragement from all levels of

government for the development of managed-care programs. The cooperative type of community care that developed in Saskatch-ewan during the Medicare crisis of 1962 (and earlier) has persist-ed. It is far from widespread across the country, but there is much interest in it. Quebec has advanced the furthest in alternative health care delivery, with a network of more than 160 communi-ty health and social services centers (*centres locaux de services communitaires*), staffed entirely with salaried medical profes-sionals and run by community boards (Rachlis and Kushner 1989:236–41).[59] Ontario has slowly begun to develop community-based health service organizations (HSOs), which are not unlike some American HMOs, except they are primarily government-funded.[60] The provincial government has also turned greater attention to the potential offered by community health organiza-tions (CHOs), which are larger managed-care organizations (not necessarily full-service facilities in and of themselves).[61] In gener-al, these alternative, clinic-type facilities emphasize preventive over curative health care and reflect growing interest in self-care, mutual aid, and healthy environments. To facilitate their devel-opment, many provinces must change certain existing regula-tions.[62] Legislation is playing a decidedly proactive role in these small but important changes, not too unlike the past when the federal government sanctioned the innovations of a few provinces and encouraged others to join.

The role of the federal government in these developments is neither interventionist nor aloof, but it is supportive when called upon. A 1986 report issued by the federal minister of national health and welfare, entitled *Achieving Health for All: A Frame-work for Health Promotion*, outlined a new focus in Canadian health care delivery toward encouraging the development of alternative facilities. Resources devoted to preventive health care, promotion of self-care, and public health have grown con-siderably but still remain small compared to the costs of the hos-pital sector. Cost control remains an important motivation, to be sure, for all levels of government. But because the Canada Health Act relegates cost considerations as secondary to the mainte-nance of universal access to comprehensive services, all levels of government are continually engaged in determining their indi-vidual and collective ability to meet each individual's social right to health care.

Cautious Integration
Between Profession and Government

Perhaps the most difficult challenge presented by the CHA was in the area of extra-billing privileges for physicians. The issue displaced any semblance of collaboration entailed in the practice of negotiating fee schedules, and reinserted a contentious political atmosphere that rubbed open the raw reality of opposing interests between the medical profession and government. With the switch in 1977 to a combination of EPFA rules and tax points, several provinces found themselves better off permitting extra billing than using the alternative of increasing compensation for physicians to satisfy their income demands. Provincial government actors had struggled to reach agreements with their medical associations on fee schedules, and many of the agreements were fragile. The ban on extra billing required by the act jeopardized several mutual understandings achieved after years of negotiations.[63]

All the provinces but one—Ontario—managed to legislate bans on extra billing by agreeing to submit disputes to binding arbitration, as suggested in the Hall Report and supported by the CMA.[64] The CHA required that if provinces agreed to use binding arbitration, the decisions of panels could not be altered in any way by provincial governments. In Ontario a feeble effort at compromise was made when physicians offered to refrain from extra-billing the elderly, social assistance recipients, and the needy. The provincial government refused to accept because physicians would still be violating the terms of the CHA. Instead, the provincial government unilaterally passed a bill in 1986 banning extra billing.

The problems in Ontario were far from settled by the legislative fiat. Passage of the legislation banning extra billing was followed by a bitter physicians' strike, which revealed tensions within the ranks as well as between the usual opponents. GPs only agreed to join the strike on the OMA's pledge to reduce the income gap between them and specialists (Taylor 1990:178). After 25 days, with no resolution in sight and with a clear loss of public and media support, the OMA called off the strike. Instead of launching a legal challenge to the Ontario bill alone, the OMA decided to join the CMA in a lawsuit against the Canada Health Act.[65] The lawsuit stalled in the courts for years. In 1990 the OMA decided to withdraw its case pending the installation of "fair and independent" binding arbitration for settling pay disputes with the provincial government. The turnaround resulted from a recognition by the OMA that both government actors and public opinion were against extra billing and that the medical profession needed to reestablish its credibility. Outweighing the baggage of positions that supported extra billing was the realization that "it is critical that the medical profession be a full partner in the management of the health care system so that damage can be minimized and viable solutions identified and implemented" (Fletcher 1990:28).

To this day, all provinces continue to allow physicians to opt out of provincial health care plans. Only in Quebec and Manitoba can opted-out physicians charge their patients above the provincial fee schedule; however, neither the physicians nor their patients receive any reimbursement. Elsewhere the provincial government reimburses patients of opted-out physicians at the fee-schedule level. Opting out has thus been rendered an ideological exercise. The arguments against extra billing, based on the understanding that provision of health care services does not represent a market situation (Evans 1983), have become well established in Canada, but not within the mainstream of organized medicine, whose leaders harbor the suspicion that the loss of extra-billing privileges "led to a reduction in their bargaining power with the provincial governments" (Deber and Heiber 1988:571). Some provincial medical associations continue to issue separate schedules to reinforce their differences with the provincial reimbursement levels. Frequent "economic updates" are published in the medical association journals as reminders of the discrepancy and to justify persistent recommendations that fee schedules be revised upward.

Yet, despite this persistent contention over domain and authority, a nascent willingness to cooperate is apparent in some areas of the profession's relations with government. Realizing perhaps the odds against them, physicians are experimenting with a wider range of alternative forms of reimbursement and delivery. For instance, entrenched as the concept of fee-for-service payment is, more physicians are now working on a salary or capitation basis. And the CMA now formally recognizes that "there is no single best method of remuneration. There should be flexibility of choice in methods of compensation . . ." (CMA 1991:5). The OMA has, as a result, felt obliged to sponsor seminars informing its members of the prospects, problems, and varied considerations they should give when accepting these alternative remunerative arrangements (Henderson 1990). As provincial governments lean toward experimenting with alternative practice settings and payment methods and as increasingly more reports criticize the stranglehold of the fee-for-service system, the profession is engaging in considerable soul-searching. For years there has been increasing dissatisfaction among physicians themselves with the fee-for-service schedules, not only because of the differentials between government and association scales, but also because of differentials among specialties and among the provinces in reimbursing the same specialty. All these discrepancies have highlighted the need to bring some additional considerations into calculations that were ruled as much by political power as by technical rationality. The medical profession in Canada has become more interested in measuring the relative value of work, and medical associations in some provinces are experimenting with variations of the American resource-based relative-value scale. As in the United States, the resulting adjustments in reimbursement are improving the compensation of general practitioners and family physicians, while other specialties are being demoted on the pay scale (cf. OMA 1991, 1992).

We can also see an openness maturing within the profession in two other issue areas: medical resource policy (including physician supply and distribution) and utilization controls. Developments in these two areas reveal changes in roles and relations between professional and government actors as both acknowledge the decreasing relevance of past practices and attitudes for solving current dilemmas in health care. They warrant fuller discussion.

Physicians as Labor

Labor resource policy in health care seeks the most efficient allocation of medical and ancillary labor for a given population. These objectives have been hindered by government ineffectiveness in controlling the training and distribution of health care labor within each province.[66] Two basic problems in achieving labor resource efficiency have been physician dominance in defining the issues and what has come to be recognized as an oversupply of physicians. The compromises and promises that were necessary to pass the Medicare legislation aggravated both of these problems by contributing to accelerated education and research opportunities, construction of more hospitals, and regularization and upgrading of physician incomes. These developments were not coupled with similar improvements for health care substitutes for medical professionals. At first it was thought that Medicare would increase patient demand and so would require an increase in physician supply, but this assessment proved incorrect.[67] Moreover, the emphasis on physician supply was not complemented by a fuller understanding of changes that are moving health care away from individualized specialist and technologically based care toward teamwork and primary and preventive care.

Nor did government policy in its early phases interfere in any way with professional self-governance and self-regulation. In essence, physicians controlled their own numbers and distribution. The evolution of governmental authority in general in guiding health care provision has strengthened the resolve of provincial government actors to control physician resources. The federal government is constitutionally prohibited from regulating this domain, but constitutional issues have become of secondary concern, for the federal government willingly assists the provinces upon request in their common goal of controlling physician supply and distribution. There is now agreement among some government actors that "Professional governance in the form of self-regulation is fundamentally ill-suited to maintain or promote the collective public interest" in health care (Lomas and Barer 1986:247). But the process of broadscale social construction of that collective public interest has only begun; it is a process requiring much redefinition, collaboration, and give and take among multiple self-interests.

Some provincial governments have taken routes that are more creative than outright intervention to achieve their goals. For example, Quebec and New Brunswick are using the "carrot" of an increase in the reimbursement fee for physicians practicing in undesirable areas and the "stick" of a reduced fee for those in oversupplied areas to exercise control over regional distribution. And interest is growing across the country in community health centers, which employ both physicians and ample nonphysician personnel on a salary basis and promote prevention and self-care.

Utilization Controls

Regular meetings of provincial and federal health ministers (which now take place formally at least every few years) have become central forums for communication and support among government actors in their efforts to exercise greater control over the medical profession and develop coherent labor market policies for the health care sector. These conferences commission studies as a basis for both provincial and, where appropriate, federal government policy recommendations (Barer and Stoddart 1992). More than once the conference has proposed that provinces not only reduce the number of places in medical schools, which are publicly funded, and post-MD training positions, but also limit the recruitment of foreign students and postgraduates. Now that these proposals have been clearly stated as a national framework in the Barer-Stoddart Report, provinces have begun to act. In 1992 the provincial government in Ontario (which controls the public university system) announced its intention to cut medical school enrollments by 10 percent (Gray 1992). Many provinces are in the process of developing such physician resource controls as expenditure caps, regulation of hospital privileges, and regional distribution of both incentives and disincentives. At the least, all provinces have begun the task of collecting data to underpin the formulation of new policies for medical and health care resources. These acts suggest the reappearance of an interventionist policy regime. Only if provincial governments act on their formally articulated understanding that there is no technically best allocation of health care resources and that resource distribution involves social choices that must be socially determined, would the force of interventionism be muted.[68]

Interestingly, while viewing the new proposals with alarm, the profession is not taking the same adversarial stance to the issue of utilization of physician resources as it took to extra billing. Chastened perhaps by past failures and recognizing consumer demand for change, the CMA's response to the 1992 proposals reiterated the "imperative to cooperate" with the government in developing "concepts and strategies for a rational approach to physician resource planning" (CMA 1992). The CMA wants to play a leadership role in the development of resource utilization policy and is contributing useful advice for policymakers.[69] A statement made in the OMA's response to the Barer-Stoddart Report may be indicative of future directions:

What has become eminently clear is the urgency required in addressing the issue of physician resources. The OMA's long-

standing "non-interference" strategy no longer serves the profession well, given the utilization clause in the [1991 OMA/
Ontario Government Framework] Agreement and the Government's ambition to gain control over costs. Times have indeed
changed.[70]

Recent efforts to develop utilization reviews have focused mainly on overservicing, a problem that intensified throughout the
1980s as physicians responded to ever tighter controls on reimbursement by increasing the number of patient visits.[71] Most provinces set up boards to review physician billings; these boards were
instructed to examine utilization rates. In a few provinces (for
instance, British Columbia) the boards that conduct utilization reviews are physician dominated; in more provinces these boards
consist of lay members and government officials. The review
boards are identifying specific cases and types of overservicing and
holding violators accountable either through utilization caps on
individual physicians, hospitals, or practices or through educative
methods.[72]

Some review boards are also venturing into broader health care
planning issues. Once again, Ontario is a case in point. To signal its
newly positive attitude toward collaborative relations with the
provincial government, the OMA in 1991 initiated a Joint Management Committee to establish and implement "a comprehensive
infrastructure that will address at the macrolevel such issues as
technology assessment and application, and optimal practice patterns."[73] Part of this joint effort to manage resources efficiently
consisted of an agreement with the provincial government on the
profession's responsibility for excess servicing. The committee
suggested that it oversee a utilization-sharing formula whereby the
profession absorbs one-half of the increase in utilization.[74] The format was accepted. It is now in the OMA's own interest to inform its
members how to avoid unnecessary billing procedures, that is, to
engage in self-regulation and moderation in resource utilization.[75]
The Joint Management Committee has also begun to broach the
issue of practice patterns, including the development of guidelines
to assist in clinical decision making. The profession's organizational leaders believe that beyond being "a very powerful tool" in
dealing with medical/technological complexity and in bringing
"order, direction and consistency" into medical practice, explicit

guidelines "will enable . . . physicians to defend themselves much more effectively against blunt approaches to cost containment, such as expenditure caps and global budgets" (Henry 1990:13). Although the comment is a reminder of past hostilities toward the whole concept of cost containment, and in particular its consequences on such indicators of physician autonomy as fee-for-service practice, it is also a recognition that physicians should seize the initiative for appropriate change to avoid having government take unilateral charge.

The attention being given to physician resources, utilization reviews, and practice guidelines is serving the critical function of offering the medical profession both a rationale and the tools to begin greater micromanagement of its own affairs. Many physicians have accepted the offer. The result embodies new roles for physicians in elaborating forms of self-governance that conform to provincial and national goals for both cost control and universal and equitable access to health care. Moreover, in accepting these responsibilities, both professional and governmental actors are exhibiting a willingness to experiment with a new order of social relations. Whether or not the foundation is enough to actually build an integrative policy regime remains to be seen.

Conclusion

The polarities of a segmented policy regime are in some ways more vivid in Canada than in Britain or the United States; its principles and norms of separate domains persistently inform roles, relations, and decision making in health care. An interventionist policy regime appeared with the passage of key legislative measures and temporarily offset the dominance of a segmented policy regime and the centrifugal forces it occasions in Canadian federalism. The Hospital Insurance and Diagnostic Services Act, the Medical Care Insurance Act, and the Canada Health Act established a role for the federal government in funding and overseeing the system of national health insurance. But the institutionalization of an interventionist policy regime was uneven, because its principles and norms were weakly spelled out by the overly general terms of the legislation. As a result, in specific matters of health care, federal government intervention seemed to return to the more minimalist level of facilitating provincial efforts, sometimes only when asked.

Government intervention in general is not as intrusive at the microlevel of health policy in Canada as in the other two countries. It is a last resort, to be used when self-governance fails to uphold national rules and regulations.

In settling long-contested issues of federal/provincial and governmental/professional rights and responsibilities, the Canada Health Act allowed experimentation with alternative forms of payment and delivery. The emergence of an integrative policy regime is discernible, but only barely, in these newer experiments being conducted by the provinces. The past has been more acrimonious in Canada than in either Britain or the United States, and so the healing process that must precede an integrative policy regime has been more tenuous and strained. But the fact that the various actors involved (provincial government actors and medical professionals above all) are beginning to engage in accommodative, cooperative, and collaborative decision making indicates that past modes of governance according to the principles and norms of segmented and interventionist policy regimes no longer fully apply to the social relations of health care. Insofar as no one regime prevails, the Canadian health care system seems to exemplify an adaptive coexistence among the three types of policy regimes. Greater reliance on an integrative framework of roles, relations, and decision making may yet emerge from more experimentation with alternative forms of health care provision.

NOTES

1. The difference is that when these experiments occurred in Canada, they tended to include more people proportionate to any given population and to be facilitated by municipal or provincial legislation, so that their impact was greater. Besides early instances of private contracts and voluntary prepaid plans, a municipal doctor system began in 1914 in Saskatchewan, whereby municipalities retained doctors on an annual salary basis. Parallel municipal hospital plans, which both fulfilled constitutional obligations to the indigent and expanded beyond welfare to include taxpayers, also began (Taylor 1990:34–37; Naylor 1986:32). These innovations spread to neighboring Alberta and Manitoba, albeit on a reduced scale. Such early experiments tended to occur in the western provinces, more predisposed to collectivist ideas because of a strong cooperative movement based there. In addition, Newfoundland, which joined the Confederation in 1949, introduced a Cottage Hospital and Medical Care plan in 1935.

2. Note once again the ironic role of Conservative governments in welfare state expansion.

3. Conditional grants-in-aid can appropriate devices for implementing social programs under federal jurisdiction. However, as in the case of national unemployment insurance, they may require a constitutional amendment.

4. After World War II federal/provincial conferences began to take place every five years in order to renegotiate tax agreements to fund Canada's expanding welfare state. They are momentous events for both the potential conflict and compromise they portend.

5. Federal actors recommended: (a) that the provinces continue their wartime agreements to forego the imposition of personal and corporation incomes taxes, and add succession duties, leaving the federal government full and exclusive access to these revenue sources; (b) that the federal government expand its present payments to the provinces according to a formula based on provincial increases in population and production; and (c) that provinces commit themselves to these agreements for a trial period of three years.

6. To make matters worse, the Liberals lost some seats in the 1945 election, weakening King's ability to push legislation through the House of Commons.

7. Although the literature generally considers the 1945 Conference a failure because it did not result in national health insurance, the alternative conception offered here is warranted in that it emphasizes the process of social construction in achieving Canada's unique form of health insurance.

8. Although the proportion of GPs fell for most of this century (in 1940 they were approximately 80 percent and in 1960 approximately 60 percent of all doctors), they now represent a steady 50 percent of all doctors in Canada.

9. The code elaborated certain anticompetitive measures, such as the following: "a rich practitioner should never give free service to the well-to-do." It advised that "as 'a point of honour' doctors 'in every town and district' should adhere to a single fee schedule" (Naylor 1986:21).

10. Legislation for health insurance came close to realization in Alberta, where an act was passed in 1935 but was never implemented because the government was defeated in an election, and in British Columbia, where a draft bill was introduced in 1935 but indefinitely postponed because of electoral losses in ruling-party strength. The prospect of legislation in British Columbia despite the strong opposition of organized medicine represented a low point in that province's medical politics. Because of Depression-era worries, physicians insisted on fee-for-service remuneration and an income ceiling for government assistance for indigent care that allowed physicians to charge wealthier patients more. The provincial government preferred a capitation system for GPs and a higher income ceiling for indigent care than the profession sought.

11. Taylor (1978:25) presents the more important of these as follows: health insurance should be administered by a commission, the majority of whose members should be representative of organized medicine; any plan should be compulsory for persons having up to a specified level of income; all indigents and dependents of insured persons should be included; contributions to insurance funds should be made by the insured, employers, and government; physicians should be remunerated by method(s) they select; the schedule of fees should be under the complete control of the organized profession in each

province; no economic barrier should be imposed between patient and doctor; the plan should be periodically actuarially approved; and a pension plan for practitioners should be provided.

12. For example, programs for crippled children, mental health, tuberculosis and cancer control began. For the full list of conditional grants in aid, see Mahler (1987:89).

13. The premier of Ontario put it succinctly: "I would prefer to stay out of [the medical field] entirely, because of the implications and the cost" (quoted in Taylor 1978:140).

14. Although by 1950 about 5.5 million Canadians had some form of hospital insurance, coverage and benefits were inadequate and the private plans were expensive, especially for those not under group plans. Three provinces (Saskatchewan, British Columbia, and Newfoundland) had government-sponsored plans. Private nonprofit (Blue Cross) or for-profit plans covered most of the insured population.

15. Always at the forefront of health care policy in particular and socialist-leaning politics in general, Saskatchewan was undergoing a smooth transition from its system of municipal, regional, and union hospitals to a unified hospital insurance system by the time of the 1945 conference. It had elected in 1944 a Cooperative Commonwealth Federation (CCF) premier, Tommy Douglas, who acted immediately on his campaign promises to reform health care. When the 1945 Dominion/Provincial Conference commenced, Douglas, who served as his own minister of health, had already set up a planning commission, had conducted a major survey of health facilities, and was ready to propose legislation to the provincial government. The aftermath of the 1945 conference validated his efforts.

16. British Columbia had experimented with several health care delivery systems throughout the century; the provincial government was willing to initiate hospital insurance but, as it turned out, was administratively unprepared. Unable to adopt Saskatchewan's comprehensive regionalized system because its population was concentrated in a small area, British Columbia set up a cumbersome and complicated system with two collection programs (compulsory payroll deductions and voluntary subscriptions). The electorate demonstrated its frustration with the system in an election that brought the Social Credit party to office for the first time. The new provincial government streamlined the system, abolished premiums, increased sales taxes, and made participation voluntary (except for those groups choosing to continue compulsory payroll deductions).

17. With the assistance of a federal grant, Frost embarked on a thorough study of provision in Ontario. The study found substantial discrepancies between premiums paid to and benefits received from all types of insurance policies. Benefits as a percentage of premiums were 85 percent for Blue Cross; 76.5 percent for commercial (group) policies; 58.2 percent for commercial (individual) policies; and 85.8 percent for cooperatives (Taylor 1978:114). The corresponding figures for premiums as a percentage of benefits were: 118, 130, 170, 116. In addition, overhead costs and unfilled need far exceeded expectations. A shrewd politician, and concerned about the costs of a transition to public insurance, Frost placed the burden of policy initiation onto the federal level. Claim-

ing that there were still too few hospital facilities in Ontario for the provincial government to undertake the obligations inherent in a hospital insurance program, he called on the federal government to fulfill its 1945 promises to facilitate provincial efforts through cost-sharing programs. In doing so he was also pushing the pendulum of federalism back to a centralized mode. His federal counterpart, the Liberal prime minister, Louis St. Laurent, was not as enthusiastic about a large federal role in health insurance as his predecessor had been. Accordingly, federal politicians were attempting to put responsibility for social policy back onto the provinces. A stalemate seemed imminent.

18. Taylor (1978:151) called the situation a "compromise," but the condition that Ontario "work without delay" to make the plan universal and compulsory was hardly onerous.

19. During the hospital insurance negotiations, nonprofit and commercial insurance companies, including the Canadian Hospital Association and the Canadian Chamber Commerce, presented their expected proposals to provincial premiers and federal representatives. But, especially with Ontario leaning toward public insurance (recall the position of Premier Frost), what little voice the private insurance industry had was seldom heard.

20. For instance, even after provinces shifted from line-item to global budgeting in the 1970s , governments could not specify areas of expenditure cutbacks, leaving these decisions to the hospital boards.

21. At their 1956 conference CMA executives offered a resolution to record favorable medical opinion toward universal hospital care, but it was defeated. Only a few provincial medical associations, specifically those in Saskatchewan and British Columbia, which had plans in effect in 1947 and 1949, respectively, appreciated that benefits from hospital insurance could accrue to private practitioners and could enhance, for instance, clinical freedom, given the greater certainty that costs would be covered (Naylor 1986:165–66). Only the Saskatchewan delegation agreed with its provincial government on the universality of hospital insurance; Ontario's delegation sided with the CMA on a personal income ceiling for government assistance.

22. The position led radiologists, anesthesiologists, and others who had been salaried by hospitals to demand fee-for-service payment. Their demands were opposed by the Canadian Hospital Association. The Ontario Medical Association extended the terms of the debate by arguing that outpatient diagnostic services should also be covered on a fee-for-service basis.

23. Although these plans varied by province, generally they consisted of an administrative headquarters within the provincial medical association that functioned as an insurance agency, collecting premiums from enrollees and reimbursing physicians. In some provinces physicians, especially GPs , were paid on either a per capita or salary basis, but most physicians were reimbursed on a fee-for-service basis at 90 percent of their fees. Thus, although the plans were service contracts, they complied with physicians' preferred method of reimbursement. Except for the 10 percent that was commonly withheld to cover administrative costs, these plans were nonprofit. In some provinces (for instance, Ontario) the medical association's plan amalgamated with other nonprofit prepayment agencies but remained under professional control.

24. The two types of plans, voluntary prepaid and commercial, were divid-

ing the market about equally, when the latter moved to seize the combative edge through consolidation. In 1959, more than 100 companies selling health insurance in Canada formed an association, the Canadian Health Insurance Association (CHIA), paralleling the physician-operated TCMP.

25. During the debate on hospital insurance, organized medicine had found support among its private-sector allies for its position that government's role be limited to subsidizing the needy. The Canadian Hospital Association had offered a hospital insurance plan paralleling the CMA's proposal for medical insurance and said that government should only fund those individuals who could not afford to join the Blue Cross plans. The Canadian Chamber of Commerce had suggested that government should support enrollment in all private plans (Naylor 1986:163–64). Although none of these alternatives was accepted, the exercise of formulating them had enabled the nongovernmental sector to articulate once again its interests in health care.

26. A national Gallup Poll taken in 1944 showed that 80 percent of Canadians approved a national health insurance plan with complete medical and hospital care provided by the federal government on the basis of monthly flat-rate contributions. In 1960 the approval rating was nearly 60 percent, even if it meant a tax increase. By 1965 the questions were becoming more specific: 41 percent approved a compulsory insurance plan, 52 percent approved a voluntary plan, and 7 percent were undecided (Naylor 1986:158, 191, 236).

27. Saskatchewan embarked on a publicly administered, universal, tax-supported medical-care insurance scheme that reimbursed physicians on a fee-for-service basis, with fee levels and extra charges predetermined in negotiations between the College of Physicians and Surgeons and the provincial government. Physicians could chose to opt out of the provincial plan and use the physician-controlled plan instead. The level of reimbursement was the same in the two plans; only administrative authority differed. The provincial government had imposed its power on the profession and offered what seemed at the time to be only minor concessions to soften the blow. In protest, most physicians withdrew all but emergency services. Since it was July many went "on vacation," some never to return. Relief doctors were recruited from Britain. Public opinion, which had been favorable toward physicians before the strike, turned negative during it. Only once before, in Winnipeg in 1933–1934, had doctors engaged in such action, and it was a much more limited protest against abuse of free medical care for social assistance recipients.

28. Moreover, the CCF, now the New Democratic Party (NDP), lost an election after 20 years in office. The medical association gloated but retreated when the Liberal Party victors endorsed the medical-care agreement.

29. All three provinces adopted their medical association's plan for recipients of social assistance and paid physicians amounts varying from one-half to full subsidization of the premiums of low-income earners.

30. In all provinces where it existed, commercial insurance was contained within a framework of regulations for minimum-service provisions, maximum allowable premiums, and renewability of contracts. By 1963 Ontario was beginning to formulate its own medical-care insurance plan based on these two types of voluntary insurance (physician-sponsored and commercial).

31. When the provincial plan first came into effect in 1963, only 21.5 per-

cent of Saskatchewan's physicians were directly billing the commission; by the time federal legislation for medical-care insurance was passed in 1967, the proportion of participating physicians in Saskatchewan had risen to 95.8 percent (Gray 1991:41–42). The reasons for this shift in support presaged the eventual acceptability of federal legislation: higher and more certain incomes for doctors under a public plan, greater ease of administration, and growing public support for public plans.

32. Originally, the TCMP had been fully under professional administration and oversight in that each provincial medical association acted as auditor of accounts and referee of service provision. But increasing competition with the for-profit market required financial adjustments. At first, physicians were willing to allow, for example, pro-rating of their reimbursement, when the survival of physician-controlled insurance was at stake. They became less acquiescent when, in keeping with the delimited revenue basis of the prepayment plans, pro-rating became a tool for imposing a ceiling (and therefore a reduction) on reimbursement. This change put the system more on a per capita basis, with little leeway for extra billing let alone fee-for-service provision.

33. Quebec had won two novel concessions in other fields of social policy: transfer of corporate tax credits in lieu of direct payments in an educational-policy matter and the right to establish its own pension plan, parallel to but independent from the Canada Pension Plan.

34. In the months of debate that followed, several important elaborations and modifications were made in the policy. The proposed federal contribution based on national per capita costs changed to one based on average costs in the participating provinces, to be recalculated each time a province entered the agreement, thereby easing the transition. The concept of public administration was relaxed so that voluntary and private insurances could administer the provincial plans, as long as they made no profit from public funds (their profits came from offering benefits outside the provisions of the provincial plans), their records were audited, and they were responsible to the provincial government.

35. It should be noted that during the first part of the period under discussion here (1971–1976), in which a new financing arrangement was being negotiated, there was actually little or no growth in health care expenditures as a proportion of GNP. However, in the year immediately before the new agreement was settled (1975–1976), the large expenditures and their rapid increases "led to the perception that health costs were unacceptably high and rising" (Van Loon 1978:456).

36. The extent of cost sharing varied by province because of the equalization formula. The poorer provinces spend only about 20 cents of each health care dollar, with the federal government contributing the remainder, whereas the wealthier provinces had to spend more than 50 cents of each health care dollar (Evans 1983). Taylor (1990:153) argues that in fact the federal government was not contributing half of the costs. The equalization formula resulted in a lesser contribution to the richer provinces; for example, in Ontario the federal contribution was 34 cents for every dollar spent on hospital care and only 18 cents for each medical-care dollar. Taylor adds that all the other provinces received less.

37. The HIDS legislation contained explicit requirements for provincial governments to license and inspect hospitals, review budgets, approve capital purchases, and collect statistics (Taylor 1978:230). These tasks were becoming less relevant and more onerous as provinces began to switch from line-item to global budgeting in the late 1960s. In addition, under HIDS certain hospital costs were not shared, including custodial-care institutions, major capital costs, direct research costs, and the costs of ancillary services (Soderstrom 1978:162). With the switch to global budgeting, which gave hospitals more leeway in their use of funds, some hospitals wished to experiment with some of these services to see if they might be more economical. The incentive to do so was lacking under HIDS and its strict accounting of allowable costs.

38. The basic tax rate was increased by two points when Medicare was enacted. In a major tax reform in 1971, the federal government decided to eliminate this "social development tax." To make up the loss to provinces, a transitional five-year Revenue Guarantee program was initiated, consisting of one tax point and its equivalent in cash to each province. But because the federal government had in effect lowered its own revenue base for its cost-shared contributions to health care and because health care costs were rising, the federal government decided in 1975 to limit the amount of its increases to the provinces for their health care costs, causing much alarm. The next federal/provincial conference in 1976 necessarily took up the whole issue of the use of tax points for funding the major social programs. Specifically at issue were the two health programs and higher education; all three were considered to be established programs and subject to periodic financial restructuring.

39. The amount was initially set at $20 per year and adjusted annually according to population and GNP increases, as was the block grant itself. The HIDS and Medicare legislation provided no specific coverage for these noninstitutional services, and the cost-sharing formula for insured services offered no incentive to provide them. Since studies were suggesting that they were lower-cost options, specifying their use seemed appropriate.

40. Most important, after the EPFA the provinces used global budgeting techniques more systematically for both hospital and physician payments, and eventually exercised more stringent control in holding down increases in these budgets. The provinces had already experienced some measure of success in controlling hospital costs, and even under the cost-sharing formula of HIDS, hospital costs rose less in Canada than elsewhere. Between 1960 and 1975 hospital costs per patient day rose 5.2 times in Canada, 13.2 times in Switzerland, and 6.5 times in France (Glaser 1980:I-10). This trend continued after the EPFA changes. Administrators in Canada were nevertheless concerned about rising hospital costs, because they were taking an internal and not a comparative perspective.

41. The Medical Care Insurance Act states, "The plan [shall] provide for the furnishing of insured services upon uniform terms and conditions in accordance with a tariff of authorized payment established pursuant to the provincial law . . . on a basis that provides for reasonable compensation for insured services rendered by medical practitioners and that does not impede or preclude, either directly or indirectly whether by charges made to insured persons or otherwise, reasonable access to insured services by insured persons" (quoted in Soderstrom 1978:131–32). British Columbia, Alberta, and Ontario

charged premiums. Insofar as premiums are a form of direct taxation, they are constitutionally legitimate for provinces. The commission devised a compromise position. They would not consider premiums as limiting access because it was employers who primarily paid the premiums. In 1993 Ontario strained the compromise by introducing an additional premium for individuals earning more than $40,000 per year. British Columbia, Alberta, and Newfoundland charged small user fees for hospitals, which were eventually banned. Most provinces charged user fees for long-term or extended-care services not covered by the legislation, and still do, because these charges are permissible.

42. This is the Breau Report, entitled "Fiscal Federalism in Canada," 1981, quoted in Taylor (1990:161).

43. One caveat: the task force felt that user fees did not necessarily bar access to health care but were contrary to the principle and spirit of the national health program (Taylor 1986:22).

44. Recall that the physician-sponsored prepayment plans regularly kept 10 percent of the reimbursement rate to cover overhead expenses, so physicians were accustomed to different rates.

45. Although the two terms are commonly used interchangeably, there is a technical difference. Extra billing refers to payments to physicians who have opted out of Medicare. Opted-out physicians charge their patients directly for the full amount of their services, and their patients pay them in full. Patients submit their claims to the provincial plan, which reimburses them at the provincial rate. Because some patients may wait for their reimbursement checks before paying their physicians' bills, opted-out physicians risk slow or no payment. Balance billing refers to opted-in or participating physicians and the difference between their charges and the provincial reimbursement. These physicians directly bill their patients for the difference only. There were variations among the provinces in the extent of extra and balance billing allowed. Alberta and Saskatchewan permitted physicians to decide on an individual-patient and service basis whether to bill the government or the patient (that is, to opt in or out) and how much. Ontario required physicians to choose whether to be entirely opted in or entirely opted out. Quebec allowed no balance or extra billing but did allow physicians to opt out and bill the patient at mutually agreed rates with no government reimbursement to either patient or physician. Thus, only in Quebec were some patients of opted-out physicians not reimbursed by the province for part of their payments. Quebec physicians had staged an extremely bitter strike in 1970, protesting these terms. They were ordered back to work, having won no concessions (Heiber and Deber 1987:64). In 1981 the proportion of doctors who extra-billed ranged from 0.5 percent in British Columbia, Quebec, and Newfoundland to 44.1 percent in Alberta. In Ontario 86.5 percent of physicans participated in Medicare in 1972 (that is, they opted in); thereafter the proportion ranged from 82 to 89 percent. Opted-out physicians tended to be concentrated in certain specialties. In Ontario, 58.3 percent of anesthesiologists opted out, 39.5 percent of ophthalmologists, 37.6 percent of urologists, and 33.8 percent of obstetricians and gynecologists. Virtually no general practitioners or pediatricians extra-billed. Also, opted-out physicians tended to practice in the more urbanized areas—60 percent in the greater Toronto spread (Heiber and Deber 1987:63–64).

46. In Ontario, for example, approximately 12 percent of physicians opted out at any one time, but extra billing only occurred in 5 percent of all accounts submitted to the Ontario Health Insurance Plan, indicating that physicians were absorbing some of the costs.

47. When determination of resource use is left to the medical profession alone, expenditures tend to escalate (Blishen 1991:121–22). In the 1970s per capita utilization rates were also increasing considerably all across the country. Lomas et al. (1989:82) estimate that between 1971 and 1985 per capita utilization rose by 68 percent, or an average of 3.8 percent per year.

48. In Ontario organized physicians managed to have this usurpation of the profession's regulatory powers repealed by the courts. A committee of the College of Physicians and Surgeons was granted control over fee monitoring; it included two laypersons and reported to the provincial plan office. It became as much an arm of the Ontario Health Insurance Plan as an independent body.

49. Taking the years 1971–1985 as a base, the figure is an 18 percent decrease in physicians' fees, adjusted for inflation (GAO 1991:5).

50. Physicians justified their demands with data showing that while physician incomes rose more rapidly than prices before 1969, they began to lag behind thereafter, suggesting a degree of relative deprivation (Evans 1983:11).

51. One estimate put the total amount of extra billing in Canada in 1981 at $54.7 million; Health and Welfare data put it at $70.28 million in 1983. These figures combine extra and balance billing (Heiber and Deber 1987:63–4).

52. Personal interview, Ottawa, May 1987. See her book (1987).

53. Under the original HIDS legislation, 95 percent of the population had to be covered. Medicare went no further. Under the Canada Health Act, 100 percent of the population was to have full access to all covered services.

54. In 1976 the Ontario Supreme court ruled that the Ministry of Health could not use the authority of the Public Hospitals Act to close hospitals for financial or budgetary considerations (Deber and Vayda 1985:452–53).

55. One must be careful about the base of these statistics. Gamble argues that the inpatient bed occupancy rate in Metropolitan Toronto hospitals has continued to grow, "with no indication of any slowdown or decrease" (1992:339). However, it is provincial policy to transport people from less-well-serviced areas to the Metropolitan Toronto area, so as to centralize acute hospital care.

56. According to an estimate made in the early 1980s, 15–20 percent of acute-care beds in Ontario are occupied by people who do not need this level of care but who must remain because of a shortage of more appropriate intermediate-care beds and alternative facilities (Deber and Vayda 1985:454).

57. These methods of control over technology mean that costlier advanced technology has tended to be scrutinized more than low technology, which is easier to absorb within global budgeting. Campaigns to raise funds for the larger items have resulted in a substantial increase in the numbers and assets of hospital foundations across Canada (Deber, Thompson, and Leatt 1991).

58. Priority is given to teaching hospitals, hospitals with large numbers of beds, or hospitals specializing in cancer treatment, but the original goal was to allow one CT scanner for every 300,000 potential referral patients. Weak poli-

cy enforcement has led to a ratio of one scanner for every 200,000 potential referral patients (Deber, Thompson, and Leatt 1991:198).

59. For a critique, see Contandriopoulous et al. (1986).

60. They are small-scale models of the British NHS in that they provide a full range of comprehensive services, including nonmedical services. Although they receive per capita contributions from the province (like the British GP system), all medical staff are employed on a salary basis (like American HMOs). Ontario's HSOs have been shown to achieve considerable cost savings in certain areas of provision. In particular, they have lower hospitalization rates, lengths of hospital stay, and drug costs than facilities in the regular system (Apland 1992:372–73). However, the Ontario government has recently become disenchanted with existing HSOs because they have not been as cost effective as originally anticipated. They have also been slow in developing preventive care and in using nonmedical personnel. Nevertheless, applications for HSOs are currently being processed at the rate of five per month.

61. They are funded by the government on a per capita basis but pay their providers on a salary or contract basis (Henderson 1990; Linton 1990).

62. For example, Ontario required that routine infant check-ups be performed by a medical doctor, but many clinics and cooperatives were finding that other health care professionals can effectively perform these services (Apland 1992:375). These HMO-like experiments are not inconsistent with the original Medicare legislation, which did not sanction any particular form of health care delivery or physician payment but simply specified that health care be comprehensive, universal, portable, and publicly administered.

63. The CHA stated that for every dollar of user fees or extra billing levied within a province, one dollar of federal funding would be withheld for a period of three years. If compliance occurred by or before the three-year limit, withheld funds would be returned; otherwise the province would lose the funds. Three months after the passage of the CHA, the federal government began withholding funds, forcing the five provinces affected to take immediate action on a sticky problem (the other provinces had already eliminated the practice). See Heiber and Deber (1987:68) for the amounts withheld.

64. These provinces would have preferred to sidestep binding arbitration in order to maintain governmental power to dictate the amount of fee increases, but their maneuverability was blocked by the bitter opposition of the medical profession to the whole issue of banning extra billing. Manitoba physicians gave up the right to opt out and to use job action in exchange for agreement to use binding arbitration in fee negotiations and disputes, much to the vehement protest of the province's Association of Independent Physicians.

65. The legal claim was twofold. First, the Canada Health Act was a violation of the constitutional division of powers between the federal and provincial governments. Second, it violated the Charter of Rights and Freedom by restricting both the economic right of physicians to contract with patients at an agreed-upon fee without state interference as well as "the right of patients to choose their own doctors if some physicians opt out of Medicare and bill at higher rates" (*The Canadian Medical Association Journal*, Vol. 134, January 15, 1986, p. 162. See also Deber and Heiber [1988:571]). The Charter was passed in 1982 to correct general deficiencies in the declaration of rights and freedoms

in the constitution. It was part of a broader set of amendments to the constitution (Mahler 1987, Ch. 3).

66. In a controversial case in British Columbia the provincial government attempted to control the quantity and regional distribution of physician billing numbers. Every physician in British Columbia must have an identification number in order to bill the province for reimbursement; in the past these numbers were granted routinely upon request. In 1983 the provincial government passed legislation to establish oversight of new numbers issued to newly minted physicians or physicians moving into the province from elsewhere. One physician who had been denied a new number sued the province in 1985 (Barer 1988). The case went through all levels of the court system until 1992, when the Supreme Court of Canada found in favor of the physician(s), stating that the legislation was a violation of the Charter of Rights and Freedoms. Without the ability to control the supply of new physicians, provincial governments now feel hamstrung in their efforts to develop and implement effective physician resource policies. The federal government controls interprovincial mobility of physicians, but through inconsistent licensure terms and procedures, which have hampered broader national goals for redistribution of physician resources.

67. It was based not on epidemiological studies but on physician-formulated forecasts (Lomas and Barer 1986:257) and goes back to the Hall Commission Report of 1964. The 1980 Hall Commission Report warned of an oversupply of physicians.

68. Modifying technical rationality with social concerns was a theme in the Barer-Stoddart Report. The medical profession responded positively (cf. CMA, "Suggested Principles for Responding to the Barer-Stoddart Report," mimeo., October 24, 1991). The words may all be rhetoric, to be sure, but it is a new and compelling rhetoric.

69. For example, in devising incentives for physicians to practice in underserviced areas, governments should consider prospects for spouse's employment and opportunities for children's education (CMA, "Suggested Principles for Responding to the Barer-Stoddart Report," mimeo., October 24, 1991:4-5).

70. Memo from Dr. Marjorie Keymer, chair, to the board of directors, December 3, 1992.

71. The OMA now has its own estimates of utilization increases. For specialists in Ontario overall utilization increased by 43.81 percent in 1984–1985 and by 48.11 percent in 1990–1991 (OMA, Reports to Council, June 1-2, 1992, p. 36).

72. Evans et al. (1989:575) observe that utilization review boards or committees "have neither the mandate nor the resources to go beyond statistical outliers in their investigations; even in this role, . . . they are not very aggressive or effective." This view may pertain to the British Columbia utilization review system, which is physician controlled, but less so elsewhere. A study of the Manitoba Medical Review Committee, which is also composed primarily of practicing physicians, found that between 1971 and 1985, despite a drop of 23.4 percent in real fees, physicians managed to increase their volume of services by only 9.2 percent per physician, a very low rate compared to other provinces. The author (Wahn 1992:724-25, 727) attributes this indicator of control to the committee's method of investigating and penalizing individual cases

of overuse, as well as to the committee's independence from professional medical organizations and to support from the government. The fact that Manitoba has fewer physicians to monitor and review also helps. For a critique of the conceptual premises of utilization review, see Peachey et al. (1992), who argue that the multiple factors contributing to overuse include technology, aging of the population, and expanded coverage.

73. OMA editorial, "Responsible Use of Health-Care Resources," *Ontario Medical Review*, February 1992, p. 1. Alberta, Quebec, Newfoundland, and the two territories have similar forms of joint management committees.

74. The agreement, which ended the stalemate in fee negotiations in 1991 with a global increase of 3.95 percent, included a general formula for utilization sharing. The provincial government pays for utilization increases resulting from population and demographic changes plus 1.5 percent; the rest is shared on a 50–50 basis. The exact figure for the utilization increase that was shared in 1991–1992 was 3.6 percent. The OMA recovered its portion by charging all its (fee-for-service) members equally. There is dissatisfaction among members about this collectivization of payment for utilization increases, and changes are expected toward more individualized penalty payments, once the method of identifying culprits has been determined (OMA, *Reports to Council*, June 1–2, 1992, pp. 7, 32–34). British Columbia, Saskatchewan, Manitoba, and Quebec also have various systems for tying negotiated fee schedule increases to physician responsibility for over-utilization (Lomas et al. 1989).

75. For example, "not bill[ing] OHIP [Ontario Health Insurance Plan] for completing requests from third parties for uninsured medical services such as employee medical and insurance company examinations" (OMA Editorial, "Responsible Use of Health-Care Resources," *Ontario Medical Review*, February 1992, p. 1).

Chapter Four

The United States

Health care politics and policy in the United States have oscillated between partial achievements and partial retreats. Several times in the last half century national health insurance seemed imminent. Renewed expectations in the early 1990s prompted searches for clues as to how the present might be different from the past. Much seemed to be the same, with the politics of contention and compromise taking center stage. Even more disconcerting, neither the spirit of reform nor the unusual conjuncture of political, social, and economic circumstances that ushered in the hallmark Medicare and Medicaid programs seemed repeatable. Nevertheless, important changes have occurred in the social relations of health care in the United States. They are highlighted in the policy regimes framework that is the focus of this study.

Since the early years of this century, social reformers in the United States have appealed to government to improve access to health care programs. World War I sparked discussions about health policy similar to those in Europe. These early efforts were easily stamped out, however, by references to German socialism. Not until the New Deal era did government respond beyond the domain of public health to consider the special health care needs of the poor. Since President Roosevelt was more interested in jobs and economic recovery, the medical provisions in the Social Security Act were modest. But they initiated discussion about the government's role in health insurance, a discussion that would remain on the public agenda and intensify. Increased congressional activity surrounding the 1943 Wagner–Murray–Dingall bill (for compulsory medical and hospital insurance for all persons covered by the Social Security Act and their dependents) waned as the nation became preoccupied with the war. But at least the theme was introduced, so that when it resurfaced under more favorable conditions it could not be depicted as radical. President Truman's unequivocal support for national health insurance stagnated in the face of postwar weariness with shortages and economic controls, and renewed activism by organized physicians and their supporters, before fading into the Cold War era, when any whisper of socialized medicine was treacherous. However, under the Eisenhower administration, several programs prepared the path for the "big bang" that took place in the 1960s (Leman 1977). With the passage of Medicare and Medicaid, government actors in the United States could no longer ignore the social responsibility of the state in health care.

That the United States even instituted Medicare and Medicaid and gradually expanded the reach of these programs, continuing all the while to progress toward an American-style system of health care, indicates that health policy has a central place in American welfare state development. The story of the evolution of health care policy epitomizes the "reluctance" of the American welfare state: Government actors entered the field warily, by a back door, and not of their own initiative, and retreated at the first whimper of protest over government intrusion. But they did not exit the field. The role of the state in this policy area has grown, albeit slowly, and moved away from an early acquiescence to professional domination and control. During the 1960s the state became an arena of conflict, both mediating the conflict and acting as a "factor of cohesion." And in mediating, the state also became one of the parties in the conflict, not only performing accumulation and legitimation roles, but also engaging in the process of formulating its own position as a state—and as a welfare state implicated in health care.

This chapter explores the changing role of the state in health care with the goal of elucidating current evolutionary potential. If the provision of equitable health care becomes more important than who does the providing, health care in the United States will come to exhibit a unique public/private mix. For most of its history, health policy in the United States has been embedded in a segmented policy regime, wherein the public sector has played a secondary role to the private sector, assisting it when called upon and allowing it to determine the main features of health care provision and policy. Gradually, however, the interest of the state in health care has matured, so that this issue has come to take on a life of its own within the state. Its significance no longer depends on its being a "rare crisis situation" (Barrow 1993:129). Beginning in the 1960s, policy developments signified the advent of an interventionist policy regime. Many features of a segmented policy regime persisted, however. I investigate whether the coexistence is contradictory or complementary and whether it is yielding to an alternative form of organizing health care.

The following discussion presents three broad phases in the evolution of policy regimes, depicting roles, relations, and decision making among federal and state government actors, on the one hand, and government and medical actors, on the other. In the first phase, preceding the enactment of Medicare and Medicaid, the federal government, the states, and the medical profession each occupied separate spheres of rights and responsibilities. A functional division of labor pertained. The federal government provided matching funds to the states for their health care programs, leaving the states to decide on program characteristics. All levels of government deferred entirely to the medical profession's preferences regarding both public and private insurance coverage, as well as its definition of health care. Consistent principles and norms of exclusive domains and hierarchical roles, structuring a segmented policy regime, allow this sweeping collection into one phase of all events prior to 1965. In the second phase, following enactment of Medicare and Medicaid, the shock of soaring increases in health care expenditures spurred the federal government to adopt more forceful measures of cost control, thereby encroaching on state-level and professional domains of authority. Federal regulatory measures included new tools of micro- and macromanagement, resulting in an interventionist policy regime. The 1980s represent a transition period in policy regimes; however, in the 1990s the next form is still evolving, and its shape is obscure. The federal government is beginning to relax its propensity to control through intrusive regulations and is acquiring the capacity to manage the overall parameters of health care provision through a mutual construction of new rules, involving proactive roles for both state governments and providers. Whether or not these activities will lead to the emergence of an integrative policy regime remains to be seen. However, it is clear that the social relations of health care are undergoing unprecedented transformation.

Inserting a Federal Role (–1965)

The early history of health policy in the United States revolves around efforts to put health care on the public agenda. Before World War II government had little to do with health care, which was regarded as a concern of the medical profession. Only when identifiable social groups were at risk or public health was endangered did government step in, usually with financial aid, and usually with less federal and more state-level involvement. This early reluctance on the part of government to be a more active participant in health care is best explained by the reigning principles and norms of separate spheres of rights and responsibilities between government and private-sector actors. However, even in this first phase, solidly grounded in a segmented policy regime, contradictions and instabilities appeared. In particular, government interventions frequently threatened to uproot established practice. Those threats were usually evaded by resort to tradition, but once government measures were introduced, they rarely disappeared.

Segmented Government

One of the major explanations in the literature for the development of welfare states is increasing centralization of government and concentration of authority at the national or federal level. Hence, the persistence of strong decentralized government units—the states and localities—in the United States is often cited as a significant factor for its lagging welfare state.[1] As in Canada, the American constitution specifies a certain division of responsibilities, both functional and fiscal, between units of government.[2] Unlike Canada, several features of American government are designed specifically to preclude overcentralized government or concentrated authority (such as the separation of powers of the executive, legislature, and judiciary). We would therefore expect the structure of a segmented policy regime to be dominant in the United States. However, the division between state and federal government roles need not in and of itself prevent welfare state development. As in Chapter 3, I adopt the position that federalism in the United States can be seen as a positive force in social progress, especially because the United States may be too vast and diverse to govern as a uniform welfare state system. For federalism to function positively, however, the federal government must adopt an authoritative and unifying role, subduing powerful centrifugal forces. In the field of health care, the federal government in the United States has been groping for decades to flesh out such a role, with mixed success. It has been constrained by deeply embedded ideological fears and inbred adherence to separate spheres of rights and responsibilities. Nevertheless, we can trace a path in the development of health care policy that highlights efforts by government actors both to overcome the constraints of federalism and to use federalism more effectively to achieve some form of health care policy benefiting all citizens of the United States. Much of this early history of welfare state development focuses on the states.[3]

The States and Health Policy

From the early days of the republic, state governments held regulatory power over private (voluntary and for-profit) insurance. Private insurance began in the United States with local clubs, mutual benefit societies, fraternal orders, and lodges offering burial, life, and casualty insurance. By the 1890s doctors began contracting with some of these associations, providing medical examinations on a fee-for-service basis, or more extensive health care for the membership on a per capita basis.[4] At first, insurance companies and benefit societies were completely unregulated, leading to much abuse and fraud. States began to develop minimal regulations in the 1850s, requiring adequate reserve funds to assure reimbursement. An 1868 Supreme Court ruling that insurance companies did not fall under interstate commerce upheld these efforts and encouraged more states to adopt regulations. Not until the 1940s did somewhat uniform laws exist across the nation.

The federal government did not intervene in insurance regulation until 1944, when a Supreme Court ruling in an antitrust case recognized that the insurance business had become interstate commerce (Mayerson 1968:20).[5] When Blue Cross and Blue Shield began in the 1930s, the states, upon request from these hybrid nonprofit insurance companies, gradually passed special legislation to exempt them from the usual state insurance laws and taxes.[6] State governments (and their lax regulations) facilitated the early growth of private and voluntary insurance. The federal government gave private insurance a boost after World War II with legislation sanctioning the right to include health insurance in collective bargaining. It also continued the War Labor Board's earlier policy of using tax exemptions to encourage employers to purchase private health insurance. Government actors considered employer-provided benefits less inflationary than such alternatives as wage increases (Fox 1986:149).

State governments also played an earlier and eventually greater role than the federal government in regulating hospitals (Glaser 1984). The federal government had jurisdiction over merchant marine hospitals and later over services and facilities in the Veterans' Administration; all other public and private hospitals were under state jurisdiction.[7] The proliferation of voluntary nonprofit hospitals in the nineteenth and twentieth centuries reflected the religious and ethnic heterogeneity of the United States. Many of these hospitals received some funding assistance from state and local governments in addition to their tax-exempt status. The turn of the century saw an increase in the number of small proprietary hospitals catering to middle- and upper-class patients who paid privately for their care. For all practical purposes, they were aloof from governmental or public-sector concerns until the post–World War II era. In the early years of this century state governments avoided intruding on hospital governance, affiliation aside. However, as state governments became more involved in regulating the licensing of practitioners, as the role of voluntary insurance for hospital care grew, and as the links between hospitals and universities intensified, government oversight increased. But in general, states did not exercise their regulatory powers over hospitals to any great extent until after World War II, and even then with little consequence until the 1960s.

The Quandaries of a Federal Role

From the 1910s a number of commissions were set up to consider federal adoption of some of the states' responsibilities, including health insurance. Early suggestions failed to go much beyond the discussion stage, however. The few bills that were introduced in Congress were restrained by the longstanding conception of the federal role as one of assisting the states in their domestic obligations. The federal role in social policy did widen beyond its nineteenth-century confines with the introduction in 1911 of matching grants-in-aid to the states. This mechanism strengthened the potential for federal leverage over the initiation and shape of social programs.[8] The introduction of a federal income tax in 1914, established for the war effort, further changed the face of intergovernmental social politics and formed the basis for questions that would arise later about the extent of legitimate federal control over monies collected at local levels.[9]

By the time of the Depression and the Social Security legislation, government regulatory activity, minimal as it was in health care, remained centered in the states. Separate spheres of authority characterized federal and state roles and relations, together with a reluctance on the part of the federal government to intrude in state activities and a concern on the part of the states to maintain their prerogatives. State governments engaged in minimally regulatory health policy-making. Yet at the same time, each level of government depended on the other for successful implementation of its responsibilities.

The Era of Social Security

The 1935 Social Security Act, built as it was on the solid soil of segmented intergovernmental roles and relations, was revolutionary in granting the federal government a new role in domestic matters, but one that barely touched established principles and norms. Despite the innovations in federal activities during this era, the Federal Emergency Relief Administration did not represent a takeover of state responsibilities; instead, it shored up what states were supposed to do, were willing to do, but were prevented from doing by economic constraints.[10] Grants-in-aid became a central mechanism of federal involvement in the New Deal programs, continuing the facilitative role of the federal government. The only special concern with health care was in Title V of the Social Security Act, which reactivated some earlier provisions for maternal and child health care. Title V also added certain categorical groups for whom random state and local support had been developing: the blind, disabled, and crippled children. With its multiple piecemeal targets, Title V thus reflected the preexisting patchwork of health and welfare programs, but it did affirm eligibility for tax-supported assistance for the deserving needy. It is noteworthy that old age insurance was considered a federal matter because of the high interstate mobility of the population, but this reasoning did not apply to health insurance.

At the same time, the Social Security Act proposed a new set of social insurance programs for a different group of deserving individuals: those who contribute to benefit programs from which disbursements could be considered as theirs by right. These programs fell within the domain of the federal government. Thus, the Social Security Act as a whole established an umbrella for the dual principles of the American welfare state: assistance to the needy as a state and local responsibility, and contributory social insurance as a right administered by the federal government. The explicit role of the federal government in state welfare programs was one of matching grants-in-aid; states could decide for themselves whether or not to participate. At this point in social policy history, the federal government exercised little of its potential leverage over the initiation and shaping of assistance-based welfare programs. In contrast, in the social insurance programs the federal role was substantial and the programs became increasingly more centralized over time, with regional offices facilitating coordinated administration. All in all, the health care measures in the Social Security Act were minimal, and health care itself was considered secondary to other, more pressing concerns, particularly income maintenance and national security. Those measures that did pertain to health care left its provision up to the states.

The consequences of the Depression for health care, together with the growing expense of hospital care, prompted President Roosevelt's Committee on Economic Security to conclude in 1937 that the "policy of leaving to localities and states the entire responsibility for providing even nominal public health facilities and services had failed in large measure" (quoted in Stevens and Stevens 1974:112). In this era, however, discussions of control over health care costs had little impact. Nevertheless, although a segmented policy regime persisted, the environment of ideas on both health care and the economy was creating an unsettling quality to state and federal roles and relations.

During the Depression, continued study of the problems in health care, conducted by various federal committees, substantiated the need for greater access to health care and elaborated the problems individuals encountered in paying for health care. Picking up on suggestions in committee reports, President Roosevelt summoned the first National Health Conference in 1938, inviting participants from the medical, social work, and related professions, as well as representatives of labor, industry, and government. The conference was followed by a series of congressional bills, some of which received committee hearings (Anderson 1968:112). While the issue of a federal role in health care was squarely confronted, the nature of that role was unclear, ranging from funding assistance to hierarchical central–state–local administration. The proposals suggested various roles for state governments as well as for private insurance companies or mutual benefit societies. No bill proposed a national health service, such as would emerge in Britain. In all the proposals, the role of the federal government in health care was circumscribed in some way, at the least by invoking the terms of the Social Security Act and its limited federal intervention in states' rights and responsibilities.

Broaching a National Program

Truman was the first president truly interested in health care as an independent policy issue, and he unashamedly advocated compulsory national insurance. However, he was never able to muster sufficient congressional support for any of his domestic programs, including health insurance.[11] With the Cold War effectively silencing voices that favored national health insurance, Truman turned his attention to special groups in need of health care. His advisors had begun urging a more focused approach for both levels of government in funding medical care for those who did not have private insurance, especially the needy elderly and welfare population. A 1950 Social Security Amendment, building on the consensus of the earlier conference, allowed states to use part of their federal grants-in-aid to pay providers directly for services for the elderly poor. But the Truman administration initiated this expansion in social provision too late to see it through any further. A bill introduced in 1952 for more coverage for the elderly poor under the Social Security Act was soundly defeated.

The Eisenhower administration, however, continued the expansion. Eisenhower himself believed that voluntary insurance should be the foundation of health care provision.[12] Building on earlier debates about extending the Social Security Act, his administration oversaw the 1956 introduction of disability insurance: income maintenance for those aged 50 to 65 who were unemployed because of permanent and total disability. Thus, a group that had been the sole responsibility of the states came under federal jurisdiction as a right. Benefits for the wives and dependents of persons in the armed forces were also reinstated, and incremental expansion of benefits to veterans themselves ensued. In addition, in 1959 Congress initiated, and the president authorized, payment of half of the health insurance premiums of federal employees, placing the federal government more in line with other major employers. Expansion in these measures revealed a momentum that tends to occur in social programs when policy statements are properly packaged to reflect prevailing predispositions and institutional arrangements. A major achievement of the Eisenhower era was, in fact, to introduce these measures without great fanfare, making them seem to evolve naturally out of established practice.

Much public attention in the 1950s focused on the health needs of the elderly poor. In 1957 the Forand bill proposed expanding health benefits to all the elderly, as a right and regardless of income or contribution, under the Social Security Act. The bill died in favor of a more acceptable middle-ground approach that melded a number of proposals made throughout the 1950s.[13] This moderate alternative became the Kerr–Mills bill, which extended the system of vendor payments to the elderly needy. It provided federal matching grants-in-aid (50 percent to 80 percent of costs) to those states that chose to participate, and it allowed states to pay health care providers, both hospitals and physicians, directly for their services according to state determinations of limits and scope of indigency and benefits. In a not unfamiliar pattern for the United States, the federal government's struggle to avoid a national program in the face of pressure to do something for the needy planted the seeds for an expansion in provision. The Kerr–Mills bill added a new category of persons to the roster of those deserving federal protection as a right: the medically needy elderly, who were poor but not receiving cash assistance. (In 1962 the blind and totally disabled over age 21 were also included.) State governments were given a veneer of self-determination, a barrage of "exhortation and advice" about participation, inadequate guidance on how to participate effectively, and a modicum of financial support if they so chose (Stevens and Stevens 1974:32). Despite the increments, the reluctance of the federal government to go beyond its traditional role of assisting the states through funding only perpetuated the framework of a segmented policy regime.

Implementation of the Kerr–Mills bill reflected and exacerbated contradictions in the separation of intergovernmental rights and responsibilities in the field of health care. While the Kerr–Mills program appeared to reinforce the notion that government in general was responsible for assistance to the needy, it highlighted the paradox of circumscribed programs, fragmented by levels of government and by groups of recipients. Kerr–Mills targeted the elderly poor; yet after passage of this reform legislation, the total proportion of elderly recipients of government assistance declined (from 14 percent to 13 percent).[14] The failure of the program to meet the needs of the elderly was blamed on the failure of the states to live up to their obligations, whether out of inability or lack of will. However, a contributing factor was the specification of separate roles, which tends to lead actors to do only what they are supposed to do. This consequence went unrecognized because intergovernmental relations were conceptualized as a fixed zero-sum game of state versus federal roles. A renewed effort to resuscitate expansion of health benefits as a right (the Forand bill reissued as the King–Anderson bill) failed to pass in 1960, but it did revive discussion of what constituted an appropriate federal role in health care. Once again questions were raised as to whether the accident of fiscal history ought to be corrected by granting one or the other level of government authority over the terms of social programs. Answers divided along partisan lines of concern about both social expenditures and intergovernmental relations.

In the early 1960s efforts were directed at constructing a compromise health care bill. Tensions were high, because of the failure of Kerr–Mills as well as the appeals of a new Democratic administration heralding health care reform. The legislation that was passed in 1965—the Medicare and Medicaid bills—added to problems in the social-political relations of health care by incorporating all points of view and all predispositions, and by calling the hodgepodge that resulted the American "system." Medicare and Medicaid offered something to everyone. Supporters of Kerr–Mills saw their pet program continued under Medicaid and extended to additional categories of the indigent as determined by states. Supporters of a compulsory national system with health care defined as a right for the elderly saw progress in Medicare Part A, which funded hospital reimbursement out of contributions to the Social Security Fund. Medicare Part A also represented an unprecedented increase in the role of the federal government, but curiously, it was confined to hospital care. National health insurance advocates were less appreciative of Medicare Part B, which was based on voluntary participation in nonprofit private insurance plans only partly subsidized out of general revenue. However, the Part B provisions appeased opponents of a larger government role in health care. The compromises also meant that what was given in any one section was modified, if not taken away, by another. As a result, Medicare and Medicaid prolonged rationalization of the inconsistencies that had accumulated in matters relating to the roles of government in general and levels of government in particular.

The segmented policy regime that structured relations between federal and state government actors in this first phase of health policy was deep-seated. And it led to a mode of decision making that relegated health care policy to issues of jurisdiction. Although there was widespread recognition of the need for a greater government contribution to health care, concerns about sources and extent of provision and about the rights and responsibilities of levels of government hindered government involvement. When action finally did come, it was confused and resulted in unanticipated consequences. Health care provision took on a life of its own in the next post-1965 phase.

Segmentation Between Profession and Government

Historically, doctors in the United States had a more disreputable legacy of quackery to live down than their counterparts in Britain or Canada. It tainted their budding quest for professionalization and created a lasting sensitivity among them to issues of professionalism and professional autonomy. Nevertheless, American doctors were exceedingly successful in achieving status and power in a short time. They also became highly politicized in order to protect their harder-won trophies. Although more immersed in political ideologies than elsewhere, professional/governmental relations

in the United States have not been as acrimonious as those in
Canada, nor as autonomous and deferential as in Britain. Medical
authority in the United States nevertheless reigned supreme over
governmental decisions about health care. The specter of European
socialism provided American doctors with a convenient tool to
keep government at bay.

Profession and Power

Early relations between doctors and government in the United
States involved the states more than Washington and consisted of
establishing the legitimacy of the medical profession as a major
player in staging health care policy. Doctors in the United States
began to organize under the banner of the American Medical Association (AMA) in 1847.[15] As part of its bid to professionalize, the AMA
asked that state legislatures license physicians, thereby initiating a
formal relationship with government. However, the AMA wanted to
control the terms of this relationship and convinced state legislatures that examining boards should be supervised by AMA physicians. The AMA's next objective, the improvement of medical education, was eased by the Carnegie Foundation's publication of the
Flexner Report in 1918, which called for a tightening of standards
in medical schools. AMA members collaborated with foundation
representatives, and the close links that were forged served the
medical profession well in establishing its separate, private sector
sphere of authority.[16] State governments supported the Flexner
Report and continued to play a facilitative role, improving medical
education according to the AMA's definitions.[17] Thus, within the
first decades of this century the AMA secured a significant measure
of physician autonomy and control of medicine. It won by default,
however, because government actors did not dispute the authority
of the profession to control medicine and displayed little interest in
playing anything more than a secondary role.

Undoubtedly, the authority of organized medicine derived primarily from the profession's knowledge claims, and this specialized authority granted the profession its reserved place in the
social relations of health care policy.[18] However, the bane of the
profession and a persistent source of the political contention that
tested its authority arose from its efforts to expand its power base
from knowledge alone to include fiduciary control of the financial
relationship between doctor and patient. The principle of fee-for-

service as a direct basis of payment by patients was established early as the prevailing mode of remuneration. But there was more to the principle of fee-for-service in the early American context. American doctors customarily adjusted their fees as they saw fit according to patients' incomes, a form of what can be called "price discrimination" (Bjorkman 1989:25). In justifying its discretionary financial powers as a method of cross-subsidization that enabled doctors to acquire sufficient income from the wealthy so they could afford to care for the poor, the profession was asserting its social role in health care. That the assumption went uncontested in the early days of this phase was indicative of the profession's authority.

However, intrusions into physicians' financial powers also came early, with the result that the clinical and knowledge-based autonomy of American physicians was muddied by issues of payment. As payment became a public issue and vulnerable to intervention, physicians' clinical autonomy was affected. The first main area in which the fiduciary claims of physicians were questioned was that of insurance. In general, political activity on insurance coverage ran in two directions: one for various forms of private insurance, both voluntary and commercial, and another for compulsory government-sponsored insurance. In its positions on health insurance, the AMA has consistently had to react to events taking shape outside of its sphere of legitimate authority. Rarely has it been able to define the parameters of the debate on insurance. From early on, the AMA may have inadvertently subjected the profession to public criticism and government intervention because of its unwillingness to divorce the issues of payment and medical expertise. In claiming that intrusion into its fiduciary relationship with patients constituted intrusion into its authority as a knowledge-based profession, organized medicine managed to delay government-sponsored health insurance. But as government intervened to ameliorate the inequitable consequences of a lack of universal health insurance, it intruded on the clinical autonomy of American doctors. In other words, segmented roles and relations between the medical profession and the government in the United States have never been clean and clear. And government intervention in the fiduciary physician/patient relationship created a contentious political atmosphere between government and the medical profession. However, intervention was less intense at first than it later became, because government remained for the most part outside the field of health care.

The Loyal Opposition

From the inception of "contract practice" in the latter decades of the nineteenth century and "corporate practice" in the early decades of the twentieth century, the AMA opposed any infringement by employers or health care entrepreneurs on the authority of individual doctors to determine medical care and maintain a fiduciary relationship with patients. Similarly invoking the slogan of "no third party" intrusion, the AMA balked at lay-sponsored health insurance, such as that offered by various fraternal orders, local or ethnic lodges, or other benefit societies as early as the nineteenth century (Starr 1982:206). Some local and county medical associations, through which AMA membership was derived, went so far as to refuse entry to physicians engaged in these insurgent types of practices.[19] Nor did the AMA look kindly on experiments in incorporating physicians into group practices, as was occurring in Oregon and California (discussed later). It was difficult, however, for the AMA to condemn those private-practice groups that were organized by physicians, especially when they were as renowned as the Mayo brothers' clinic in Minnesota. Instead, the AMA chose to emphasize the importance of individual practice in maintaining professional autonomy, and it stressed that doctors not be involved in profit-making ventures. The AMA's pristine insistence on the virtues of solo or small group practice gave room for criticism of unsupervised practices and recommendations for more comprehensive clinic-based care.[20] Not until 1959, in a bow to the reality of prepaid plans, did the AMA endorse these alternative corporate forms of insurance. It adopted a policy that "reaffirms our fundamental faith in the principle of freedom of choice, but . . . also recognizes the patient's right to select the type of medical care he wants—including a closed panel plan" (quoted in Campion 1984:191).

The notion of compulsory health insurance first gained currency in the United States in 1914, when the American Association for Labor Legislation (AALL) pressed for coverage for wage earners and their dependents. The AMA initially supported the AALL insofar as the idea of government-sponsored health insurance promised more regular payments. But as public discussion of government health insurance grew, the AMA and the state medical associations began to express their disapproval of any intrusion into physician-controlled payment, interpreting it as an infringement on the fiduciary doctor–patient relationship. Thenceforth, all suggestions of compulsory or government-sponsored health insurance or benefits were vigorously opposed by the AMA—except where the indigent were involved. The AMA's ambivalence about government support (depending on ability to pay) would provide the wedge it so assiduously sought to repel.[21]

Another wedge occurred in the field of hospital insurance. The spread of hospital plans in the 1930s forced the AMA to reverse its earlier rejection of voluntary health insurance, as long as plans were confined to hospitals and were of the indemnity, not prepaid or service, type.[22] However, when Congress was preparing in 1942 to introduce legislation for compulsory insurance, the AMA decided to endorse both Blue Cross and Blue Shield, as appropriate forms of prepayment plans for both hospital and physician services, even though only the latter was physician controlled. Its concessions became useful in its opposition to the compulsory-system proposals that were to follow under the Truman administration. In fact, the AMA's postwar support of voluntary insurance led to another reversal: to parry compulsory insurance the AMA had endorsed by the 1950s all forms of voluntary insurance, and adopted the slogan "The Voluntary Way Is the American Way" (Campion 1984:162). Against societal demands for government-sponsored health insurance, the AMA had insisted on professional control over all such endeavors, but it yielded when concessions could forestall legislation or influence terms of agreement. The implicit threat of more intervention loomed constantly, making the modus vivendi of a segmented policy regime unusually precarious in a country so attuned to the virtues of separate domains.

Postwar Concessions

One major area of consensus between government and professional actors was the need for growth in the supply of medical care. Yet once again, because of the AMA's initial resistance to divorcing the issue of clinical autonomy from its control over the economic factors of supply, consensus on the broad issue did not enhance its power base. Instead, another wedge for government intervention inadvertently opened when the AMA did finally yield. The AMA could not help but support the Hill–Burton Act of 1946, which authorized a huge increase in federal funding to states for hospital and clinic construction. Additional legislation expanding federal funding for biomedical research at medical facilities, as well as at the National Institutes of Health and the newly created National Science Foundation, was also noncontroversial. But when the notion of supply of medical resources was applied to physicians themselves, the AMA protested. From its early quest to attain and maintain the highest quality of medical education, the AMA has sought to limit the number of physicians trained and certified. In the early 1950s, after the first flush of Hill–Burton expenditures increased other supply and demand factors, studies were showing a physician "shortage." Yet the AMA continued to argue that insofar as physician output was itself increasing with technological advancement, more physicians were not needed.[23] The AMA eventually agreed to support increased government funding for medical education on the condition that no government intrude on academic freedom.[24] During this period, fear that the money giver might become the power wielder was overtaken by the feeling that one should not "look a gift horse in the mouth."

By the 1950s when state governments were increasing spending on education in general as part of the GI bill, medical school enrollments had swelled. There was a certain expediency to the AMA's backing of government's role—increasing expenditures on education and the resulting growth in the supply of physicians would "make medical care more accessible [and reduce the] clamor for national health insurance," some leaders of organized medicine believed (Fox 1986:193). They were joined by diehard government advocates of incremental growth in services as a better national strategy for health care than government insurance. Thus, a powerful national consensus formed in favor of increasing expenditure on health care. The consensus led, however, to an expansion in government's role in health care.

The Final Battle

During the 1950s interest had grown in Congress for measures to provide medical care to retirees through Social Security. The Forand bill for hospital and surgical insurance coverage for retirees under Social Security was introduced in the House of Representatives in 1957. The AMA, revitalized by a more politically astute administration at its Chicago headquarters and by the introduction of dues, sensed the renewal of a threat to its control. For the first time, it turned to creating a political action committee at the national level to pursue its interests (Campion 1984:210).[25] However, whereas the AMA had managed to counter earlier threats effectively through ideological appeals that were appropriate to the times and temper of American society, by the late 1950s the debate over health insurance and health care was taking on a new dimension in its focus on the elderly.

Truman had been astute in narrowing general health insurance to the elderly. As Marmor (1973, Chapter 1) notes, public support for this kind of program easily followed when data showed that the elderly were poorer and sicker than the rest of the population. But disagreement arose as to whether all the elderly should be covered, or only those who had contributed to Social Security, or only those who were financially needy. The AMA did not respond well to these social concerns. It offered no policy position, but instead hammered home its earlier positions that physicians should control decisions about medical care and that physician–patient relations should remain sacrosanct. Its statements contributed less to perpetuating separate physician and government domains than to clarifying the distinction between expensive hospital care (in which government had a mounting interest) and regular visits to doctors for nonurgent care (which doctors could fully control). The distinction had policy implications.

With the paltry results of the Kerr–Mills measures (for state-level medical care for the elderly indigent) and a new Democratic administration heralding greater access to health care, a plan to provide health care for retirees as a right under Social Security reappeared in 1961 as the King–Anderson bill. It provided for hospital insurance only, because hospital care was becoming inaccessibly expensive. In his response to this bill, the AMA president articulated a principle that would inform AMA opposition for the next several years: The proposal "compels one segment of our population to underwrite a socialized program of health care for another, regardless of need" (quoted in Campion 1984:256). The AMA's campaign to counter Fedicare, as it called the King–Anderson bill, introduced the nonprofit, voluntary, bipartisan, unincorporated American Medical Political Action Committee, formally created in 1961 in step with the inauguration of President Kennedy. It also thereby introduced a more sophisticated political arm for organized medicine, which up to then had been somewhat clumsy in its public activities.[26] Because the King–Anderson proposal did not have sufficient congressional support, especially within the House Ways and Means Committee chaired by the powerful conservative Democrat Wilbur Mills, who preferred the earlier bill that bore his name, it died a quiet death. The AMA was given more credit than warranted for this failure, probably because President Kennedy vented his frustration against Mills by attacking the AMA (Marmor 1973:53).

Buoyed by its political success but concerned about its public image, as well as about lingering dissent within its rank and file over its recalcitrance on a number of issues, the AMA continued to work with politicians to articulate measures that would ease burdens of payment and access for the elderly poor. Tax credits were a favorite panacea. At its 1964 annual meeting, the AMA went so far as to declare support for the principle that *"everyone in need, regardless of age,* is assured that necessary health care will be available" (quoted in Campion 1984:272, italics added). Without fully realizing it at the time, the AMA was voicing support for an extension of Kerr–Mills to what was to become the Medicaid program. The AMA's formal proposal, called Eldercare, offered comprehensive hospital and physician care for the needy elderly financed through general revenues. It was used to oppose what was coming to be called Medicare (the King–Anderson bill that failed in 1960 and was reintroduced in Congress in 1964). Two representatives (Curtis and Herlong) introduced Eldercare as a competing bill in the House in 1965. Since some Republican leaders blamed their party's abysmal results in the 1964 election on its association with AMA opponents of Medicare, they felt the need to formulate a position that would dissociate them from the AMA's Eldercare proposal (Marmor 1973:63). The Byrnes (Republican) bill for voluntary enrollment in a plan that included physician services and prescription coverage (it became Part B of Medicare) was thus presented—at an unexpectedly opportune time when Representative Mills could use it in a compromise. Although the resulting passage of Medicare and Medicaid signaled a defeat for the AMA, the organization's role in health politics became a significant factor in the next phase of policy development.

The AMA's initial failure to prevent the passage of legislation establishing a circumscribed right to health care should not be seen as detracting from the sophisticated level of politicization achieved so quickly by American medicine. It used its power to maintain whatever semblance it could of respect for separate domains. The dominant role of physicians in defining health care was clear, and government basically acceded to the demands of the medical profession. As we will see, although the AMA lost the battle regarding the adoption of legislation, it was very influential in specifying many of the details of the new programs. However, relations between government and medical actors remained wary. Every step in policy development was viewed by physicians as an attempt to intrude, confirmed at last in 1965. Thus, the principles and norms of a segmented policy regime structured contention as a modus vivendi between government and medical actors. Even though "most elected officials tried to avoid confrontation with organized medicine" (Fox 1986:158), the demands of health policymaking superseded. The appearance of a full-fledged interventionist policy regime in the next era legitimated and expanded government's role in health care.

Testing the Regulatory Waters (1965–1981)

The principles and norms of separate domains are ensconced in the American Constitution and are fundamental to American political values. At the same time, however, the wars and economic upheavals of the twentieth century subjected segmented roles and relations to constant testing. Not until the convergence of political and social factors in the 1960s did the supporting base for a segmented regime in health care policy seem to collapse—"seem to," because the illusion of change brought about by Medicare and Medicaid was more apparent than real. Although the legislation portended a new structure of governance, change was incremental, chipping away first at the economic viability of the old framework before setting up the foundations for a new policy regime. Segmented roles and relations, deeply embedded in state/federal relations, persisted alongside new measures through which the federal government attempted to regulate the activities of state government actors. However, an interventionist policy regime more readily structured professional and governmental roles and relations, as the norms supporting segmentation lost ground to the demands of the economy.

Intervention: Federal on States, States on Providers

The Complexity of Medicaid

After passage of the 1965 legislation, health policy transactions between the states and the federal government were confined to the Medicaid program. Medicaid left most of the previous problems of welfare medicine intact. A functional division of responsibility seemingly granted authority to the states with the federal government subsidizing program delivery, much as before. The authority of the states was derived from their wide latitude in determining eligibility and services. This role was somewhat encumbered by the language of the legislation, which declared that states should provide for groups of persons ranging from the "categorically needy" to the "noncategorically related medically needy" (Stevens and Stevens 1974:61). Most states translated these terms to mean that, beyond what they were already doing, they could add new groups of recipients as they saw fit. In a similar vein of delegated but unclear authority, states were required to provide five basic services, beyond which they were free to expand as best they could to achieve a system of "comprehensive care."[27] Although one could characterize the goal of comprehensive health care as expansionist (Stevens and Stevens 1974:Ch. 4), in practice the Medicaid program was vague about its purposes in providing health care. The act of providing, rather than any sense of outcome, guided the states. Indeed, programs that were "below minimum standards of health and decency" were funded without punishment or incentive (Stevens and Stevens 1974:78). Substantive purpose in the Medicaid program focused on its welfare function, which, in the United States, separates one specific group from mainstream society and restricts its access.

Also unclear was the extent to which the federal government would act beyond its traditional funding role or use its fiscal powers to actually improve health care. Where the possibility of a stronger federal presence did exist—in guiding, directing, or overseeing state programs—the federal government more often than not fell back on its traditional role and simply assisted the states financially.[28] Little more leadership was forthcoming. The availability of funds was considered to be sufficient encouragement for states to embrace their constitutional responsibilities and provide health care for the needy (Vladeck 1979:535). However, the expectation of adequate health care was contradicted by an assumption of cost containment. Because states had to contribute their share of funding, it was assumed that they would endeavor to control costs. But again they received no guidance as to how. In addition, unanticipated additional costs occurred because Medicaid's welfare population had costly health care needs, including emergencies. Although states had discretion in principle in distributing Medicaid largesse, pressing needs reduced the value of state flexibility.

One of the goals of the original Medicaid legislation was to encourage states to accept the terms of the program and to undertake circumscribed health care provision to the best of their ability, and this was met. All the key indicators of provision increased— from number of states participating, persons benefiting, services offered, and of course monies expended. By 1967, however, when Medicaid had reached less than half of the program's original intended population and was far from providing the full range of comprehensive health services, the unexpected cost increases resulting from success led to a reconsideration of Medicaid's goals. The rapid rise in Medicaid expenditures was particularly shocking because this program was for a welfare population. (It should be noted that Medicaid expenditures increased at a much smaller rate than Medicare, but the latter program enjoyed more public support.) But the means not the goals, expenditures not health care, became the focus of concern.

The interpretation used earlier to place blame for the failure of the Kerr–Mills program—incompetence on the part of the states—was renewed, and its invocation at this time laid the base for the regulatory thrust of an interventionist policy regime. Changed conditions could no longer support a shoring up of segmented roles and relations. Instead, the federal government used its power of the purse to exert control over the states. More specifically, Congress issued an increasing array of regulations that states were to follow in their dispersal of cost-shared funds. The first major change occurred with the passage of the Social Security Amendments in 1967, clarifying the categories of persons eligible for Medicaid by specifying income level.[29] These amendments also clarified the nature of the mandatory benefits and limited the federal role in encouraging expansion.[30] Although the original five mandatory services remained intact, requirements for achieving "comprehensive care" were relaxed even more. Thus, at the same time as the federal government was delimiting its role, it was also constraining the states' financial and administrative capacities to fulfill their obligations as set out in the original legislation. These regulations exacerbated problems in providing for a welfare population. As a result, the federal government became more directly involved in state-level responsibility, beginning a vicious cycle of inadequately correcting errors, which led to more errors, and more attempts at correction.[31] Each new series of Social Security Amendments throughout the 1970s continued this trend of specifying eligibility and service criteria, and in so doing, reining in the reach of the Medicaid program.[32] And yet, despite increasing restrictions, expenditures increased unrelentingly.

This advent of regulatory politics, insinuating as it did that errant states required corrective direction, inserted intrusive federal measures intended to change state behavior. But these initial ventures into regulation were ambivalent, insofar as they invaded the constitutional division of responsibilities and established assumptions of a separation of spheres. The results were therefore erratic. Moreover, the Medical Services Agency in the Department of Health, Education and Welfare (HEW), which was to be the federal agent of regulatory control, was not yet sufficiently developed as an institution to offer the broad direction required. Accordingly, this introduction of an interventionist policy regime exhibited a typical liberal welfare state penchant for micromanagement, which tends to occur in situations of ambiguous goals, limited means, and unclear bases of authority, and which makes the force of intervention deeper than intended.

States and Hospitals

The federal government's efforts to control state expenditures through micromanagement represent one face of the interventionist policy regime that began to emerge during this era. It also had another face, a mirror image in which state government actors asserted their power vis-à-vis one of their main counter-actors: hospitals. By the late 1960s, several states had become critical of the federal government's vapid leadership in controlling hospital costs, and so they began to exercise their own fiscal and legislative powers over hospitals. Federal government actors responded with encouragement for these state efforts. As states engaged in hospital regulation, they began to acquire the capacity to take a firmer stand against hospitals' spending desires and to follow through on their interests in controlling costs. Thus, the interventionist policy regime in this area exhibited a characteristic politics of contention over different understandings of what constitutes adequate health care.

Early steps toward a new system of governance were awkward in the American context of revered separate domains. The states first exercised regulatory control over hospital expansion.[33] Their individual efforts were unified by the 1974 National Health Planning and Resource Development Act, which mandated the certificate of need (CON) program. CONs were the basis of broader state planning efforts and required that institutional capital expenditures of $100,000 or more be reviewed first by regional Health Systems Agencies, and then approved by state planning agencies. This hierarchical edifice was to result eventually in centralized planning and regulation at the federal level, but the scaffold of federal guidance on the activities of planning agencies was bare. Accordingly, although the new construct portended a transfer of authority from local to federal levels, and thereby raised considerable objections from doctors, nothing of the sort materialized. The federal government continued to delegate authority over difficult decisions— above all, denying expenditures—to state and local levels. To ease the pain of such power, the legislation establishing CONs gave the states and their planning agencies considerable latitude in determining priorities and in choosing the representatives on agency boards.[34] The resulting loose and pluralistic regulatory framework defies easy assessment, but to the extent that generalization is possible, studies showed that CONs and Health System Agencies did not contain costs (Benjamin and Downs 1982).[35] But we must add that at this point cost control was simply a hope. This early effort to control hospital expenditures was more important as an exercise in a new type of roles and relations, based on improving the regulatory skills of state actors. It was a much larger task than states had undertaken before, and one that would not succumb readily to imperfect mechanisms.

Another area of increasing state control over hospitals was rate regulation. Under the 1965 legislation hospitals were to be reimbursed for "reasonable" costs under the Medicaid program. A few pathbreaking states, finding that their increasing expenditures to hospitals were anything but reasonable, began to regulate per diem rates.[36] Concern about hospital rates was occurring in the private sector as well.[37] Therefore, recognizing that controls were imminent, state hospital associations collaborated with state legislatures to write the legislation and guide the staff in state agencies. Eventually, utilization of hospital services also came under investigation, and the arsenal of regulatory tools available to state governments expanded. Throughout the 1970s a number of states were reviewing hospital utilization under the Medicaid program, using a variety of methods to identify, for example, unusually long hospital stays, to broach the subject of unnecessary surgeries, and to contend with these. The experiential and data bases for later regulations that began during this era continued throughout the 1970s and into the 1980s, as more states adopted some form of hospital rate regulation and utilization review. States began to acquire the technical capacity to exercise their legislative power and deny hospital requests for expenditure increases.

These early efforts to develop CONs, hospital rate regulation, and utilization reviews were initiated by the states. The federal government reinforced and encouraged the states, sometimes by joining the various strands of regulation under an umbrella, as in the 1972 Social Security Amendments. But for the most part, the federal government focused its own efforts in another area where its responsibility was clearer: Medicare and physician fees. Thus, this introduction of an interventionist policy regime was uneven for federal/state roles and relations but clearer for state governments and providers.

Government Intervention in Professional Domains

The AMA took its failure to prevent the passage of Medicare and Medicaid as a defeat for organized medicine. The soul-searching that followed resulted in a rejuvenated and more sophisticated level of politicization. Up to the 1960s the AMA had been using fear of government regulation as a harbinger of socialism to maintain the status quo of professionalism, claiming physicians could deliver quality care only without interference. After the 1965 legislation, the AMA effected an about-face. President Johnson and his staff at HEW, whether out of pragmatic recognition that successful implementation of the new legislation rested on the full cooperation of physicians, or because government was unprepared, bureaucratically and politically, for the newness of the federal role implied in the legislation, invited the AMA to help formulate rules and regulations for Medicare and Medicaid. The AMA welcomed a new, seemingly more constructive role—though, by becoming such a willing partner so soon, it infuriated some diehard rank-and-file members. But the benefits realized dissolved any disharmony. A new working relationship was established between organized medicine and government; rising above past confrontations and accusations, the two sides now cooperated, each offering constructive suggestions for change mindful of the concerns and interests of the other (Campion 1984:280–81). However, the prospect of collaboration was tenuous.

Worries About the Foot in the Door

A central area of contention involved physician fees under government-regulated programs. Some of the terms in the Medicare legislation, particularly in Part B, which covered payment for physicians' services, had acceded to physicians' interests.[38] For instance, physician (and patient) participation in Part B was voluntary.[39] And Medicare reimbursement was based on the principle of "customary, prevailing, and reasonable" charges, an acceptably vague standard with little technical meaning. Notwithstanding these favorable conditions, physicians' fears of government control led them to raise their fees across the board. Between 1965 and 1967 physicians' fees doubled, twice the rate of increase in the Consumer Price Index (Marmor 1973:86; Campion 1984:325).

However, the medical profession's attempt to maintain financial control backfired. Because inflation was more pronounced in health care than in other sectors of the economy, President Nixon continued the wage and price controls of his 1970 Economic Stabilization Program on all physician fees and hospital charges for two additional years (limiting annual increases in the former to 2.5 percent, the latter 6 percent). Further, hoping to allay unstabilizing consequences of future growth expected in Medicare, he proposed, and Congress accepted, an increase in Social Security taxes, softened by a counterproductive increase in benefits. When the controls were lifted, a very disgruntled medical profession raised its fees with a vengeance, from a growth rate of 3.1 percent in 1973 to 12.5 percent in 1975. But in the same year the "customary, prevailing, and reasonable" basis of reimbursement was modified for the first time with a more exact formula, the Medicare Economic Index, which limited increases in fees by a measure of changes in practice costs (PPRC 1992:12; Epstein and Blumenthal 1993:195). Government intervention had become very real indeed. It is, of course, ironic that a Republican president reinforced the power of regulatory measures.

Added to the profession's travails were the persistent efforts of Congress to pass more legislation expanding health care coverage. The AMA's focus was deflected from payment issues to initiatives coming from a coalition between organized labor (particularly the United Auto Workers) and key senators (particularly Edward Kennedy). Organized medicine could at first do little more than react to these developments and endeavor to keep the forces of change under control if it could not actually prevent their realization. By 1969, however, an increasingly more pragmatic AMA leadership accepted the principle of health care as a right and led the organization toward the kind of positive, constructive stance with which it had weathered the previous legislative onslaught. The AMA countered renewed congressional interest in national insurance with a proposal for graduated income tax credits covering the purchase of health insurance premiums for those still without adequate coverage. The program was called Medicredit; the AMA clung to the idea throughout the 1970s .

Indirect Intervention Through Review Processes

In another instrument of control over physicians—medical reviews—federal government actors attempted to coopt physicians in order to mitigate the sting of intervention. Since physicians at first successfully adapted the tactic to their own interests, it took many years for reviews to become powerful tools of micromanagement. The original Medicare and Medicaid legislation included provisions for two types of government oversight responsibilities: (1) certification of hospitals meeting minimal quality standards and (2) utilization reviews, including general reviews of the quality of physician practice patterns and specific reviews of resource use. It should be noted that the government was not trying to exercise technical control over physicians or hospitals. Government deference to medical authority was initially guided by the expectation that with minimal government regulations in place, health care providers would begin to exercise self-control of their practice and expenditure patterns, so that government monitoring would no longer be necessary. As for quality control, the AMA had no problem with proposals for quality assurance insofar and as long as the task remained under AMA control (it was already one of the organization's several educational activities). Because of the profession's opposition to greater specification of the terms of utilization reviews, which implied external controls, the Social Security Administration set up a convoluted and diluted system that basically left such reviews in the hands of physicians at the hospital level. Insurance agency intermediaries were empowered to conduct claims reviews under the Medicare and Medicaid programs, but without enforcement powers.

As it became obvious that these mechanisms were not working to control costs, both the legislative and executive branches of government suggested strengthening their effectiveness through more active physician involvement. In response, the AMA proposed Peer Review Organizations (PROs) as an extension of an already well-established process of peer review on technical matters in hospitals. By this time (the early 1970s), however, government actors wanted more, especially more assurance that all hospitals would establish well-functioning, well-organized reviews, and that costs themselves, not simply technical-medical matters, would be the central objective of review. Congress, in short, wanted a system of internal audit. Thus, the 1972 Social Security Amendments transformed the PRO concept into Professional Standards Review Organizations (PSROs), stating that their goal was the promotion of "effective, efficient and economical delivery of health services of proper quality" (quoted in Campion 1984:328). In this way the federal government embarked on the arduous task of imposing its authority over the activities of physicians. Repeating a scenario that had followed the passage of Medicare and Medicaid, the AMA leadership bowed to reality and helped translate the legislation into workable terms of implementation, angering once again those rank-and-file members who remained unconvinced that any benefits could result from such overt government intrusiveness.

By 1974 HEW began funding over 200 PSROs. These early peer reviews focused mainly on factors in hospital utilization, especially length of stay. One significant contribution of PSROs was initiating movement away from a retrospective reimbursement approach by instituting concurrent reviews of utilization requests. In addition, some PSROs developed profiles of individual physicians and began advising and monitoring those who had, for example, more than the normal number of hospitalized patients or patients with unusually long hospital stays. Thus, the idea that individual practice patterns and decisions could be externally scrutinized was gradually introduced by physicians themselves, albeit under government pressure. Nevertheless, despite an Office of Professional Standards Review in Washington and the attempt to introduce federal government scrutiny of issues of quality and practice as they affect cost, PSROs remained physician-dominated, operating according to locally determined standards.[40]

With the creation of the Health Care Financing Administration (HCFA) in 1977, an explicitly unified approach to control over health care funding commenced, intensifying physician concern over federally directed reviews. HCFA began by assisting regional PSROs to develop standards and norms on which to base assessments, conducting pilot projects to test the effectiveness of a number of alternative forms of cost control, and engaging local practitioners, providers, and researchers. Reacting to fears about an ominous future, the AMA began to advocate replacing PSROs with a voluntary review program. Since congressional evaluations of PSROs were indicating that they had minimal effect on costs, and since the mood that was to usher in an era of deregulation was already present by the end of the Carter administration, plans were initiated to phase out PSROs.

The PSRO program and its consequences represent a turning point in medical politics. Senator Wallace Bennett (Republican), who introduced the PSRO legislation, envisioned this program as a last opportunity for the medical profession to take control of quality and costs before someone else did (Bjorkman 1989:56). Congress had repeatedly told the AMA and other groups in organized medicine to develop a solution to rising costs, but the profession produced no cost containment strategy whatsoever. As a result, organized medicine lost political clout, its expressed concerns overtaken by the overriding problem of rising health care costs. The solution that emerged in the next phase of health policy—prospective payment to hospitals according to Diagnosis Related Groups (DRGs)—emanated from an agency, HCFA, prepared to offer a sharp technical bite to any new legislation. It brought to a head years of ineffectual government attempts to exercise control over physicians and their contribution to rising health care costs. And it thereby fully instituted the interventionist policy regime that had been building for years in these preparatory regulations.

The Social Politics of Incentives (1981–1992)

Although the Reagan presidency heralded a new era in American politics, in the field of health care it brought about a fruition of initiatives begun earlier. Despite the rhetoric of deregulation, regulatory government became fine-tuned and therefore more powerful. However, during the 1980s regulation changed from the micromanagement that had characterized government intervention in the 1970s to a macromanagement that masked its deep interventionism. This era consolidated an interventionist policy regime in health care at the same time as it introduced hints of alternative social roles and relations.

Loosening Federal Intervention

President Reagan's call for a "new federalism" harkened a return to traditional segmented roles and relations between federal and state levels of government. However, Reagan also wanted to define the federal role more clearly, and in particular to limit its reach and to rein in its tendency to go beyond established boundaries. A favored method, which he had used as governor of California, was to set caps on expenditures; this smacked more of intervention than the segmentation and separation favored by conservatives. Although the president was not able to get Congress to accept his proposals for caps, variations on the theme did materialize.

Reagan's first effort at targeted cuts for the Medicaid program occurred with the Omnibus Budget and Reconciliation Act (OBRA) of 1981. This statute called for federal Medicaid contributions to be reduced each year by a steadily increasing percentage. It also eased some of the restrictions on state calculations of eligibility for Medicaid, which resulted in a decrease in the number of recipients. The OBRA 1981 cuts were combined with a new block grant system that excluded Medicaid, but set the stage for further reductions in the interventionist role of the federal government. The symbolic implications of the block grants proved to be greater than their financial consequences. They conferred considerable discretion on the states, but offered them little incentive to spend less money and little assistance in coping with reduced federal funding (Bovbjerg and Davis 1983).

State Initiatives

Throughout the 1980s the states took the initiative in engaging in new methods of cost control, strengthening their regulatory power over providers. Whether their efforts were the result of the new tone of federalism under the Reagan administration or were undertaken out of frustration with the federal government's laggardness is debatable and probably not generalizable. Several states continued to improve their hospital rate setting and utilization review techniques to the point where studies found substantial expenditure reductions that could be directly attributed to the stronger state efforts.[41] In their continuing endeavors, several state governments were becoming more innovative, relying not only on established regulatory techniques but also on provider cooperation.

One major indicator of innovativeness on the part of some states occurred in their increasing requests for waivers from federal regulations governing the Medicaid program (Dobson, Moran, and Young 1992).[42] Among the waivers requested were those seeking to loosen the requirement that Medicaid patients maintain free choice of provider. Successful states began to experiment with managed care and with greater use of home and community services instead of nursing homes. Although states interpreted the waiver process as a roadblock, the federal government encouraged their efforts more than it thwarted them. Compliance with certain regulations is the intent of the process.

Despite the Reagan administration's call for deregulation, a few states stepped up their efforts to control hospital costs. An underlying thrust behind these initiatives was movement away from multiple payers and retrospective reimbursement toward a more integrated all-payer system.[43] All-payer systems went far beyond any earlier state efforts to consolidate insurance programs. They attempted to streamline the different rates paid by different types of insurance carriers (rates were especially disparate between group or employer-based plans, on the one hand, and payment by individuals, on the other); to eliminate the many bilateral agreements reached between Blue Cross plans and individual hospitals; and to impose some semblance of fair price if not fairness in the payment system. Exposed to public view for the first time were hospitals' clandestine methods of price discrimination as well as the entire insurance system's cost-shifting affronts.[44] States adopted various methods of setting insurance rates (Maryland set up an independent commission, New York a new state Department of Health) and accommodated different patient populations and hospital needs in various ways. The measures thus reflected different state priorities and politics. With a few exceptions, the all-payer system has been successful in those states where it was initiated (Thorpe 1993).[45]

In this era, federal government control over the states receded, but state government control over providers increased. To the extent that states undertook the initiatives out of frustration with both providers and the federal government, a politics of contention reigned. However, insofar as the macromanagement tools being developed were more cooperatively based and less intrusive than earlier measures, state efforts were precipitating the construction of a new order in the social relations of health care, as we shall see.

Consolidating Intervention in Professional Domains

Congress had wanted to consider a prospective payment system for Part B of Medicare at the same time as the Diagnosis-Related Group (DRG) formula for Part A was under review, but was dissuaded by AMA opposition.[46] Following the enactment of the 1983 DRG legislation, Congress asked the Department of Health and Human Services (DHHS) to study and develop an appropriate plan for cost containment in physician and medical services. After some stalling in the executive branch, the DHHS delegated the job to HCFA. At the same time, Congress pointedly raised the urgency of the issue by freezing physician payments under Medicare in 1984 and asking both the Congressional Budget Office and the Office of Technology Assessment to conduct studies on physicians' fees. In 1986 HCFA formally commissioned a group of academics and physicians at Harvard who had already been working on a new methodology for calculating a resource-based fee schedule. The Harvard group collaborated with both practicing and research physicians to develop the scale. A first report was presented to HCFA in 1988.

Meanwhile, Congress appointed a new agency, the Physician Payment Review Commission (PPRC), to advise it on further Medicare reforms.[47] The PPRC began by arming itself with its own data and studies and was prepared to review the Harvard team's first report immediately. Its review process was purposely open and included consultations with physicians and beneficiaries as well as public hearings. In 1989 the PPRC recommended for congressional approval a slightly revised version of the Harvard team's fee schedule.[48] OBRA 1989 enacted the results of this political-bureaucratic process of revising physicians' fees. The Medicare Fee Schedule commenced its phase-in period in 1990 with full implementation beginning in 1992. Completion is expected in 1996. On the surface it was a major extension of government regulation, one that firmly established an interventionist policy regime in physician/government roles and relations.[49] At the same time, however, the fruition of this interventionist policy regime may contain the seeds of change. Whether one characterizes the fee schedule as a highly interventionist form of regulating physician payment and by implication physician behavior, or a rational appeal to rise above politics and understand the objective reasons for prices depends on how one characterizes the role of physicians in the formulation of the schedule and in the changing social relations of health care. The case for interventionism is self-evident; the case for nonmarket and nontechnical rationality needs elaboration.

Physicians were ready for a change in the "customary, prevailing, and reasonable" form of reimbursement. They were not, however, ready en masse to give up fee-for-service reimbursement. The PPRC therefore considered a relative-value fee schedule a less radical form of physician payment control than either capitation or a DRG-type of service package (Oliver 1993:137). The AMA has consistently expressed approval of a resource-based relative-value scale (Ginsburg 1989; Epstein and Blumenthal 1993). In addition, the purposeful consensus-building work of the PPRC, as well as its concern that physicians understand and accept the changes in payment it engendered, rallied support.[50] This is not to belittle either the profound aversion that exists among some physicians and their intense protests to the fee schedule, or the split within the medical profession on methods of influencing improvements in the fee schedule. It is to note that concessions have been made all around to the fact that new rules must structure a new game, and to the realization among physicians that if change does not occur through cooperation, it will occur some other way.

Substantial changes were estimated in Medicare reimbursement to physicians based on the fee schedule. Some procedures (evaluation management and primary care services) received increased payments of over 30 percent compared to past "customary, prevailing, and reasonable" payments; others (surgeries) decreased payments of 30 percent (see PPRC 1990:xiv). By the time the Medicare Fee Schedule was implemented in 1992, considerable backtracking on a number of items reduced the full impact of the decreases. Nevertheless, further study and recalibrations are continuing. Unless there are future reversals, the consequences of the fee schedule for the social relations of health care, if not necessarily its costs, could be revolutionary—especially if it moves beyond the scope of the Medicare program alone, which is not unexpected.[51] To the extent that physicians appreciate that the schedule is an improvement over the previous payment system, one that may aid their faltering public image, and to the extent that physicians continue to be involved in recalibrations of the schedule, the medical profession may be putting itself into a more collaborative relationship with the government. Some physicians, individually and in organized groups, are attempting to work with government actors to achieve the cost control that all seek. They continue to remind government actors of the unique role of physicians in health care, but they are more willing to absorb some losses for the sake of a mutually agreeable understanding of a broader concern about the outcome of health care. And they are trying all the while to adjust to a seemingly inevitable diminution of medical dominance in health care.

In addition to the issue of fees, government actors are testing their relations with the medical profession in another, formerly sacrosanct domain of physician autonomy: physicians' individual decisions on whether to participate in the Medicare program (known as *assignment*).[52] The first federal government attempt to use financial incentives to encourage greater acceptance of assignment by physicians in the Medicare program occurred with the Participating Physician and Supplier Program, a subset of the Deficit Reduction Act of 1984.[53] In addition, Medicare was to publish and distribute directories of participating physicians. The proportion of claims made on an assignment basis increased from 55.8 percent in 1983 to 68.5 percent in 1985 as a result of the program; this was the first major increase in the assignment rate (PPRC 1989:359).

Legislation passed in 1985 began, gently, to limit the completely open-ended scope of physician choice in accepting assignment.[54]
With the introduction of the Medicare Fee Schedule came the need
to strengthen these regulatory mechanisms to prevent a decrease in
assignment and an increase in extra billing. Accordingly, in 1989
the PPRC recommended that unassigned charges be limited to a
fixed percentage of the fee schedule payment.[55] It also explicitly
recommended against mandatory assignment at that time
(1989:136–37). There is no doubt that these measures represent
encroachments on physicians' freedom to choose assignment, even
though neither the incentives nor disincentives are unduly harsh.
What is more important, however, is that the framework within
which these new policies are being developed is unlike what one
would expect within an interventionist policy regime; for example,
because physicians are not excluded from decision making. And,
while their interests and concerns are integral to policy outcomes,
physicians do not dominate (as they would in a segmented policy
regime). The same can be said for the interests and concerns of government actors. Cost control dominates the agenda, and yet it is
not necessarily being realized in policy outcomes. It seems to be as
important to government to achieve a new working relationship
with the medical profession.

Back to Basics or
Forward to Collaboration? (1992–)

Preparing for Integration: State Initiatives

By the 1990s the states were more clearly both crying out for leadership and assuming it themselves. The number of states undertaking some manner of health care "reform" burgeoned and a typical American problem—too much variety, too little real choice—
threatened to destabilize more comprehensive system reform.
President Clinton's proposals at first offered the prospect that state
initiatives might be coordinated under a common umbrella.
Indeed, the plan relied on the states to be active coparticipants in
reorganizing and rebuilding the nation's health care system. But
legislative politics deflated expectations. Nevertheless, certain key
states plod on. Although their experiments revolve around cost

control goals, many states are venturing to extend their concerns to include universal access. Some of the more innovative states are engaging in various combinations of regulation and incentives, and in doing so, they are pulling away from governance within an interventionist policy regime to experimentation with principles and norms more characteristic of an integrative policy regime. I briefly review a few state-level accomplishments in passing and implementing several of the goals in President Clinton's original and now moribund plan for national health care reform. The cost savings achieved in the state-level plans are, for the most part, explicitly intended to provide universal coverage.

Some of the state experiments have required Medicaid waivers; these have mainly been for health maintenance organization (HMO) demonstrations and are discussed in Chapter 5. Other experiments have required waivers from the nettlesome Employee Retirement Income Security Act (ERISA) of 1974, which gives the federal government regulatory power over employer-provided benefits, leaving regulatory power over insurance companies to the states. As more employers have become self-insured, they have become exempt from state laws. Without ERISA waivers, therefore, state innovations have only affected small employers (generally under 50 employees). By December 1994, 44 states had passed some type of small-group health insurance reform, primarily for guarantees that small employers can renew their plans without major premium increases (except under unusual circumstances), guaranteed portability for previously insured people who are changing employers, and guaranteed issue of insurance to any small group that applies (PPRC 1995:206).

Only one state has an active employer mandate program. Hawaii passed legislation in 1974 (before ERISA prevented such programs) requiring employers to contribute at least 50 percent of an employee's premiums. As of 1991, part-time employees who work at least 20 hours a week are also covered, contributing at least 1.5 percent of gross income or half of the premium, whichever is less. A program initiated in 1992 establishes a purchasing pool for Medicaid recipients and other low-income people. Hawaii is also encouraging the use of HMOs by Medicaid recipients.

Washington and Oregon have both passed legislation requiring employers to pay at least 50 percent of an employee's premiums. Implementation of these programs awaits federal waiver approval.

Washington's four regional, noncompeting, nonprofit, and voluntary health insurance purchasing alliances are among the best established in the nation. The state's Health Services Commission defines a uniform benefit package and maximum premiums for the alliances. It also sets health plan certification rules and creates service effectiveness and other advisory committees (DiIulio, Nathan, and Kettl 1994:20–23, 30–31). The state of Washington is a forerunner in requesting federal permission to integrate Medicare, Medicaid, and several other federal programs.

In 1992 California's state legislature passed a proposal enabling businesses with fewer than 50 employees to purchase insurance through a voluntary purchasing pool. It enrolled nearly 80,000 people in its first 18 months of operation (PPRC 1995:212). Employers contribute 50 percent of the premiums and enrollees are encouraged but not required to join an HMO. The California Health Insurance Plan has been successful in offering competitively priced premiums, while enforcing community rating, based on geography, age, and family structure but not health status.

Florida's plan is based on a managed-competition model. It created 11 regional Health Purchasing Alliances (state-chartered regional cooperatives) to broker the best options available for employer-based health care coverage. Employers with fewer than 50 employees are encouraged to participate, voluntarily. The Florida plan also encourages enrollment in managed-care programs. The efforts of some in the state to expand coverage in these purchasing alliances to uninsured persons who are not receiving Medicaid failed in 1994. But, as in other states that have seen recent setbacks (Massachusetts, Vermont), local groups intend to keep trying.

Another state that actively promotes managed competition and the managed-care programs it fosters is Minnesota. After passing its plan in 1992, Minnesota began phasing in basic coverage for low- and moderate-income persons ineligible for Medicaid by subsidizing the premiums of those earning less than a certain income. The plan specifies that insurance premiums cannot exceed 12.4 percent of family income, thus setting the basis for the broadest-based "community rating" in the nation. Employers are encouraged to buy insurance from a purchasing pool. One additional innovation in Minnesota is its use of tax increases on cigarette sales and on the gross revenue of health care providers (a 2 percent tax on hospitals, doctors, and dentists; 1 percent on HMOs). Kentucky,

Ohio, Rhode Island, and Tennessee have also recently undertaken programs to expand coverage to previously uninsured groups through managed-care programs.

Although four states have enacted full community rating, New York is the only state that has implemented it (PPRC 1995:208). Legislation limits variations in insurance premiums among individuals and small businesses in the same region. The system creates two risk-sharing pools: One transfers money among health plans, the second transfers money among those plans with enrollees who have specified high-cost medical conditions (PPRC 1994:141). New York has also taken the lead in combating insurance discrimination, passing legislation to prevent insurance companies from denying or limiting coverage to individuals on the basis of age, sex, health status, or occupation.

Another form of risk pooling has occurred in some states (nearly half) that have opened their state employee benefit programs to other public employee groups, such as those working in public education (PPRC 1995:213). A few states (Minnesota, Missouri, Vermont, and Washington) have permitted certain private-sector groups to join as well. These initiatives are presenting an important model for the federal employee benefits program.

Oregon's experiment has been singular and provocative. The state's plan (first enacted in 1989 legislation) involved a radical reorganization of past coverage practices under the Medicaid program. After considerable study of the state's Medicaid expenditure patterns, the Oregon Health Services Commission, composed of health care professionals and consumers, decided that certain medical procedures that had been uncritically reimbursed under Medicaid were not cost-effective. The commission prioritized over 700 treatments and decided that only the top 587 should be reimbursed. The savings from denying payment for the remaining procedures were to be used to expand Medicaid coverage to the uninsured. In 1992 the DHHS declined Oregon's request for a 5-year demonstration project waiver, indicating that considerations in the quality-of-life factor discriminated against the disabled. After making appropriate changes and enlarging the pool of reimbursable procedures, Oregon's plan was approved in 1993. More than any other state, Oregon has brought to national public attention the questions and dilemmas of scarce resources that will confront health care policy-making into the next millennium.

The exasperation with federal stalemates that propelled states to initiate their own efforts may suggest a reversion to a segmented policy regime in federal/state relations. However, if the next stages in the national policy debate continue to affirm state initiatives, as has been the case thus far, and go so far as to base national policy on state efforts (as occurred in Canada), then the terms of a segmented policy regime would be inappropriate to capture evolving relations in health care. These recent state efforts also smack of some features of an interventionist policy regime, especially with regard to government/provider relations. An important difference from past practices is that state governments are now engaging in more collaboration with providers and constructing mutually agreeable goals, which include not only cost containment but also universal access. Considerable discussion and testing of public opinion has preceded legislative moves (as in Oregon) (Brown 1991); in some states (California, for one) items are put to the ballot for approval. Since 1994 HCFA has required public involvement in Medicaid demonstrations. Whether or not any of these developments will lead to the emergence of an integrative policy regime depends on federal support of the activist states and federal prodding of the laggard states. Little will change if the federal government responds with little more support than it has offered in the past—giving states broad authority to solve problems but within restrictive guidelines (Brown 1994:156). The states are offering the federal government a unique opportunity to follow their lead. They have presented sufficient groundwork that could readily be coordinated—not only specific measures, such as employer mandates and purchasing alliances, but also breakthroughs in social relations, involving the sanctioning and motivating roles of government. Through its granting of waivers, the federal government appears to approve of the innovations in individual states, which is an important and necessary preliminary step in a federal system. The next step, however, is to integrate these experiments into a cohesive framework.

Incipient Integration Between Profession and Government

The federal government has become more proactive in its relations with the medical profession. As during the 1965 legislative inroads, in the 1980s all government actors realized that the success of renewed efforts at cost control would require the cooperation of physicians. Unlike the earlier period, however, by the late 1980s government actors became intent on bringing physicians around to a form of cooperation established more by public-sector actors than by physicians. Political experience, not deference, dissuaded officials from the distasteful intrusiveness of past government measures and led them to search instead for a new working relationship with health care providers. It is possible that the groundwork for collaboration is being cautiously laid in the new initiatives. I briefly examine two new policies, volume performance standards and practice guidelines, for further clues on assessing a possible evolution in policy regimes. A primary consideration is how adamantly the government is upholding cost containment as the fundamental goal of any new developments (as opposed to the lesser position of collaboration in evaluating cost control as well as other goals) and how adamantly the medical profession is opposing cost control (or recognizing its reality and the need for accommodation to achieve it).

Volume Performance Standards

From the beginning the PPRC appreciated that the Medicare Fee Schedule alone was insufficient to contain costs. The commission first proposed expenditure targets, but the idea was resisted by the AMA, ostensibly because expenditure targets "could force restrictions on medically necessary services" (Woolf 1990:1813). As alternatives the PPRC recommended Volume Performance Standards (VPS) and practice guidelines. These were supported by the profession as "more prudent strateg[ies] for curbing the delivery of inappropriate services."[56] The VPS and practice guidelines ideally work in tandem, representing the macro- and microdimensions of resource management tools. As such, they could be interpreted as falling within the framework of an interventionist policy regime. However, as these methods of cost control are being implemented, an unprecedented level of cooperation, suggestive of an integrative policy regime, is guiding professional/governmental relations. Although these developments are occurring only in the Medicare program, they could be providing an experiential base for broader changes in the social relations of health care.

The VPS, as specified in the 1989 OBRA legislation, is a targeted rate of growth estimated on the basis of inflation, changes in the number and age composition of Medicare beneficiaries, changes in technology, evidence of inappropriate utilization of and reduced access to necessary services, and other factors judged appropriate by the secretary of HHS. The VPS is a macromanagement tool for guiding aggregate expenditure growth that is thought to avoid past errors of intrusiveness because it is a global yet substantively based estimate and because its incentives are directed at collective physician behavior. It contains clearer bases for targeted expenditure growth than earlier measures. At present, there are several standards, each pertaining to a category of service (for example, surgical; primary care). The PPRC has recommended the development of a single standard with changes linked to projected growth of real gross domestic product (GDP) (PPRC 1995:58).

Speaking on behalf of a wide governmental constituency, the PPRC expressed the hope that when physicians compare a calculated (VPS) target with actual growth, they will clearly see the difference and realize that the difference puts physicians as a group at risk.[57] The medical profession would thereby have a "collective incentive to foster approaches to cost containment" (PPRC 1990:27). Annual updating of the Medicare Fee Schedule is now based on the difference between the VPS calculation and actual expenditures.[58] Although the commission foresees a continuing and firm federal government role in implementing the cost containment goals of the VPS, it has voiced optimism that the medical profession would "take the leading role in changing the way that physicians and patients think about using medical resources" (PPRC 1990:27). Veiled threats could be read into these remarks, but such an interpretation distorts the significance of the changed context in which physicians and government actors are working together to achieve a collective goal.

Practice Guidelines

Government actors turned to practice guidelines as a way of involving physicians more directly in cost containment, allowing them to construct their own, appropriate responses to new government regulations and the incentives and directions implied. Along with the VPS, OBRA 1989 created the Agency for Health Care Policy and Research in the DHHS to sponsor the development and dissemination of practice guidelines, clinical standards, review criteria, and performance measures in both the public and private sectors.

These guidelines are to be used for general educational purposes (for both providers and patients) as well as for payers' assessments of appropriate utilization and effective practice. Many new guidelines are being developed in both the public and private sectors and much study of their use and usefulness is underway. As a result, the new agency is also to function as a central depository and clearinghouse for dissemination and evaluation. In addition to their educational and, eventually perhaps, clinical functions, practice guidelines could form the basis of reforms in adjudicating medical liability (PPRC 1995:325–27).

There is nothing new or unusual about practice guidelines themselves; however, the involvement of a federal government agency is a radical departure. The significance of the new agency and its work derives less from its actual functions, which are minimal, than from its larger context. The process of developing practice guidelines is, arguably, the most collaborative we have seen yet in the field of health care, involving government actors, medical professional organizations, hospitals, academic medical centers, health plans, public and private research organizations, and malpractice insurers. The PPRC foresees an important federal government role in encouraging, guiding, and coordinating the involvement of private-sector actors in the practice guideline process (PPRC 1995:391). It is clearly a continuing and expanding, not a diminishing, role. The several activities involved in developing, disseminating and using practice guidelines are far from problem-free. But through engaging in these processes, public and private actors are deciding, collectively, whether cost control alone is the chief goal of reform or whether something else, such as knowledge or mutual self-help, is also desired.[59]

A series of articles in the *Journal of the American Medical Association* (Eddy 1990) suggest a future direction for practice guidelines. The author compares a traditional approach to practice guidelines, in which clinical judgment and intuition are deemed sufficient because interventions are few and straightforward, with unnamed new approaches, which recognize that practice guidelines must now inform physicians about the increasing number and complexity of choices, as well as about the costs and benefits of interventions in situations of profound uncertainty. If we could generalize, we might hazard the thought that some, at least, within the medical profession do not see the development of practice guidelines as counter to their interests (cf. Woolf 1990). Those interests have become more complicated. Questions of economics in medicine are now thoroughly intertwined with ethical considerations in which physicians need as much guidance as anyone else. These perplexing dilemmas cannot be solved through technical means, nor through appeals to medical criteria alone. It is not unimaginable, and it may even be useful, to consider these developments as events precipitating the construction of a new, integrated policy regime informing more interdependent roles and relations between government and the medical profession.

Conclusion

The hold of a segmented policy regime is strong in the United States. It is evident in the failure to achieve national health insurance and universal coverage. It is also reflected in instances of continuing government submission to physicians and other health care providers, whether as private actors or well-organized interest groups. However, alongside this traditional separation of domains, government actors in the United States have constructed a formidable interventionist policy regime. Federal micromanagement of the role of states in the Medicaid program and federal regulation of both hospital and physician reimbursement under the Medicare program assailed assumptions about autonomous domains. Recently, many health care actors have come to understand more clearly the critical role of government in general, and the federal government in particular, in health policy-making. Government's role includes regulation, but it now goes beyond the negative preventive powers of intrusive measures to such proactive measures as support and encouragement to do more. Although cost control was an initial motivation for changes in the role of government, the goal of an overall reduction in costs is being modified by concerns about redistributive equities in health care. To the extent that these conjectures are valid, they suggest a new policy regime, which I have called integrative because of the blurring of boundaries it connotes. Only tendencies toward this policy regime exist at present in the United States. Although they are largely the result of unanticipated consequences, they are nevertheless acquiring a force of their own and pointing to a new direction in the social relations of health care.

Any attempt to generalize about any area of policy in the United States must acknowledge opposing forces. Vocal and substantial groups of physicians, patients, business leaders and politicians remain adamantly adverse to innumerable specific features of changes both ongoing and impending in American health policy. At some point, however, a social scientist must stand back and try to assess the whole scene. What stands out when one adopts a historical analytical perspective are the novel roles, relations, and modes of decision making among the main actors in health care. Government actors are no longer either deferential to the medical profession or determined to impose externally derived changes in behavior. They want change, but they also recognize the value of internally derived criteria. For their part, physicians (on the whole, or at least, those who are having an impact on policy development) are no longer as antagonistic to "the other side" (that is, government). They recognize that the practice of medicine is greatly altered, with each decade bringing more complexity and uncertainty than physicians alone can manage. The norms guiding the new world of social relations and policy development in health care are no longer those of the past. To suggest that they can be captured by the term integrative policy regime in contrast to segmented and interventionist regimes is to use analytical frameworks to reveal social features that may not otherwise be altogether obvious.

NOTES

1. Thompson (1986:68) quotes Theodore Lowi as saying: "federalism is the most important single factor" accounting for the "nonoccurrence of socialism in the United States."

2. The Constitution granted the federal government authority over those functions that constituted the national interest, interpreted as national security. All other functions, understood as domestic, rested with the states. Thus, anything to do with trade and the military, including care of merchant seamen and veterans, fell under federal jurisdiction. Care for military personnel expanded in World War II to include the Emergency Maternal and Infant Care Program for wives and dependents of servicemen. Disbanded in 1947, it was replaced in 1956 by health care provisions in the Servicemen's Dependents Act. In the early nineteenth century most public health concerns were still local matters, and were taken up by the states only gradually as the problems came to be seen as more than mere nuisances. The discovery of bacteria and vaccinations brought control of communicable diseases back to local levels (Anderson 1968:19, 130). Some public health concerns (epidemics) were considered interstate and therefore federal matters, insofar as they affected trade. Care of

the needy—individuals so designated because of indigence or such specific disabilities as mental illness or blindness—rested with the states. The only exception to this division was facilities and services for Native Americans, which have always been a federal responsibility, insofar as the territories involved were interstate.

3. Various welfare state programs developed in the United States at the level of the states, or in some cases at county or even local levels. Except for their inconsistency across the nation, they became viable counterparts to the nationally administered and financed programs unfolding in Europe in the early years of this century. Workers' compensation is a case in point. In 1885 Alabama was the first to adopt legislation placing the legal burden of compensation for work-related injury or sickness on the employer; Massachusetts passed similar legislation in 1887. As employer liability proved inadequate, state government assumed more responsibility for setting up funds (Anderson 1968:58). By 1910 most European workers received benefits for injury or disability; by 1915 workers in 30 American states were covered, and by 1920 coverage had been extended in all but six states. The American Association for Labor Legislation (AALL) was a major impetus behind the introduction of these laws, functioning as the equivalent of organized labor in Europe. (The AALL was not a labor organization, but a group of intellectual, academic, and progressive social reformers, including some labor leaders and physicians.) After its initial success with workers' compensation legislation, the AALL actively pushed for compulsory state-level health insurance. However, all of the bills introduced in the 1910s failed (Fox 1986:19). Reforms in old age assistance were also undertaken by state governments. By 1930 over half of the states had pension laws in place. Similarly, such innovations as "mothers' pension" for widows at risk in caring for their children began at the state level in 1911 (Skocpol 1992).

4. The proportion of care provided by these fledgling insurance companies was small compared to the organized care offered by certain large employers and other corporate forms of delivery (Starr 1983:206–207).

5. Earlier charges of antitrust violations, as in Oregon in the 1930s, were dismissed (Starr 1983:205). Congress reinstated insurance company exemption from federal antitrust regulations in 1945 by passing the Insurance Regulation Act and the Uniform Trades Practices Act, which measures defined and prohibited "unfair methods of competition or unfair or deceptive acts or practices" (Mayerson 1968:24).

6. Among other things, the Blues are exempt from maintaining the same high reserves as insurance companies. In all but two states (Vermont and New Hampshire), the Blues are overseen by state insurance departments.

7. The distinction between public and private hospitals in the United States has been much more vague than in any other area of health care. In the eighteenth and nineteenth centuries former almshouses evolved into public hospitals, either municipal or county, but many of these relied on charitable donations for support. The only strictly state hospitals were mental institutions.

8. Federal aid programs to the states evolved from an early eighteenth century form in which land grants were administered by all levels of government: "national policy was to use public land to aid the states, with the states and

local governments assuming a role in carrying out national policy" (Dommel 1974:11). By the nineteenth century the federal government was attaching more conditions to the aid (particularly evident in education—the curriculum of land grant colleges had to contain agriculture and mechanical arts), but these conditions were still broad guidelines. Cash grants, made more frequently by the end of the nineteenth century, carried stricter requirements, and the grants themselves, including federal power to withhold them, became tools for coercing states to undertake or modify programs. Categorical matching grants as the foundation of the fiscal relationship between states and the federal government in social policy solidified with the passage of the Sheppard-Towner Act in 1922. Under Sheppard-Towner the federal Children's Bureau dispensed grants to states for a specified purpose: maternal and child health services for the poor. Insofar as these services were strictly a state function, the program was administered by the states in accordance with federal guidelines, which in this first health care program were minimal. The Sheppard-Towner Act was discontinued in 1929 as the Depression absorbed federal concerns about social expenditures. The Act's demise was also facilitated by the AMA's official disapproval of it (Anderson 1968:91).

9. Eventually the division of tax fields became inequitable, with state resources from sales taxes growing slower than federal income and corporate tax sources, while the states were still expected to provide matching grants for federal assistance. The problem was first addressed during the Depression through equalization formulas.

10. The Federal Emergency Relief program ended after two years with the installment of the Social Security Act in 1935.

11. One successful exception was early passage of the (Hill-Burton) Hospital Survey and Construction Act in 1946. Truman assembled a National Health Conference in 1948, but it came to no position on the strong proposal for national health insurance made by Oscar Ewing, secretary of the Federal Security Agency. Prevailing opinion put faith instead in the continued expansion of voluntary insurance to fill gaps in health care coverage for workers, leaving government to provide for the needy. The chair of a follow-up commission explicitly stated the issue: "We have recommended Federal grants-in-aid to these [training and construction programs] and other necessary activities because we believe that the role of the Federal Government is to stimulate them, not to control them" (quoted in Anderson 1968:127–28).

12. In his first term Eisenhower introduced the notion of reinsurance: "that the federal government with its great resources could insure high-risk and low-income groups normally not able to buy in the prevailing insurance market" (Anderson 1968:143). Since opposition to the principle was widespread, it did not pass a congressional vote.

13. The Eisenhower administration's alternative to the Forand bill was shelved; it proposed a new federal–state program of subsidy to private insurance to protect the low-income elderly against the cost of long-term illness, using a national means test of eligibility and specifying the level of benefits (Stevens and Stevens 1974:28).

14. This is not altogether unusual in the history of the American welfare state. After passage of the Equal Pay Act in 1963, women's pay as a proportion

of men's declined (from 62 to 59 percent). In most cases loopholes in liberal welfare state legislation allow for "gaming" the system.

15. Since the 1960s, when state medical associations no longer required concurrent membership, the number of American physicians belonging to the AMA has declined to less than 45 percent. Nevertheless, the AMA's positions are usually taken to be representative and it remains a relevant political actor.

16. Fox (1986:38) makes the interesting observation that philanthropic foundations in the United States played a similar role to that of the civil service in Britain, with "expert" reports and advice that informed policy developments.

17. Many hospitals also accepted the AMA's recommendation that only graduates of class A medical schools should receive internships, and state governments accordingly agreed that only graduates of class A medical schools should be allowed to take certification exams.

18. Still, in 1932 a Committee on the Costs of Medical Care, set up jointly by a number of foundations and initially endorsed by the AMA, criticized the medical profession for continuing inconsistencies in the competence with which health care was provided across the nation.

19. Between 1905 and 1917 state court rulings specifically prohibited corporations from engaging in the commercial practice of medicine, affirming the separate and widespread authority of the medical profession. These rulings did not, however, apply to "contract medicine," that is, employers hiring company doctors, nor to for-profit hospitals. Oregon and California were exceptions. In 1917 Oregon passed a Hospital Association Act allowing the incorporation of hospital associations, which hired their own doctors and offered their own insurance plans. In 1932 a county medical society in Oregon formed a corporation of physicians to compete with the hospitals, followed in the 1940s by the statewide Oregon Physicians Service. The hospital association challenged the legitimacy of the physicians associations claiming restraint of trade, but courts ruled in favor of the physicians (Starr 1983:204).

20. As in the 1932 Report of the Committee on the Costs of Medical Care; see note 18.

21. Labor leaders were also consistently wary of a paternalistic government role under compulsory insurance, thus reducing support for such a measure. Interestingly, labor was united with employers in this position. Employers, in fact, were one of the first organized groups to express support for voluntary (private-sector) insurance. Nevertheless, by the 1920s it was apparent that the earlier quest for workers' compensation had superseded demands for compulsory health insurance, and the implementation of workers' compensation temporarily satisfied demands for further social reforms.

22. Under indemnity plans patients pay doctors directly and are then reimbursed (usually in part) for their expenses by insurance companies. After World War I and especially as the Depression years advanced, the number of employers and individuals purchasing voluntary private insurance grew. By 1934 the AMA felt compelled to explicate once again its position on voluntary insurance, issuing ten principles that highlighted the central role of doctors in specifying medical care and the full terms of their fiduciary relationship with patients (Starr 1983:299–300).

23. When the AMA's own economists began to revise their methods of calculating the relationship between quantity of physicians and other factors of production and demand, the AMA was prepared to change its tune.

24. The AMA's full turnabout on the issue of physician supply did not occur until after the passage of Medicare and Medicaid; in 1967 the Board of Trustees officially announced a change in AMA policy on government support for increased medical education (Campion 1968:242). By then, however, the issue of supply was no longer a celebration of improving quality through expansion, but a zero-sum game of competition for scarce resources.

25. The 1946 election saw the AMA's first authentic forays into political activities as well. The organization had set up a Washington office in 1943 after losing an important antitrust case in the courts, and its new quarters became a base for active lobbying and campaigning on behalf of candidates sympathetic to its positions (Campion 1968, chap. 13).

26. This period saw one of the first major splits in the ranks of the AMA. A small (100-member) group calling itself the Committee of Physicians for Improvement of Medical Care was less significant than the drop in membership (by nearly 25 percent between 1946 and 1952), which was a protest against the public display of partisanship and Cold War rhetoric by spokespersons for the AMA (foremost among them the firebrand anti-Communist Morris Fishbein).

27. On the surface, the five basic required services (inpatient hospitalization, outpatient hospital visits, health clinic visits, lab and x-ray services, skilled nursing facilities) could constitute comprehensive care. But because states were free to impose their own limits (for example, on lengths of stay and number of visits), comprehensiveness was compromised. (This is an important factor distinguishing the delivery of these required services from those in Britain and Canada). Only the wealthier states expanded beyond the basic requirements to provide a full range of services, leaving a typical demarcation across the nation in treatment of the welfare population.

28. For instance, although the open-ended funding arrangements encouraged expansion, the federal government offered no guidance on how the states should expand provision. The federal government specified its own role: it agreed to provide matching funds, ranging from 50 percent to 83 percent depending on per capita incomes in the states, for their Medicaid programs, as well as an additional 75 percent for administrative costs arising from a state's need to hire additional medical personnel and 50 percent of other administrative costs. Also specified were a number of conditions that states had to meet to receive these funds; none of them was onerous, so micromanagement at this early stage was minimal. Some of these conditions, such as that the program be in effect throughout the state, were already established under the Kerr-Mills legislation; others, such as "proper and efficient operation," were perfunctory. The incentives in the Medicaid program were too weak to overcome laggard commitments by some states to their domestic obligations (Thompson 1986:648–49).

29. The means test for Medicaid was tied to the level of eligibility for cash assistance in each state. A further restriction was that federal matching funds would not be available for persons whose income was more than one-third

above the state's limit for cash assistance. This meant that in many states those who had been categorized as "medically needy" but did not meet the financial criteria were ineligible for Medicaid until their medical bills brought them down to one-third above the poverty level. One concession to the medically needy dissociated them from the rest of the welfare population: when they became eligible for Medicaid, they were paid directly for their medical expenses. For welfare recipients, state administrators (fiscal intermediaries) reimbursed providers directly (Burwell and Rymer 1987).

30. As a follow-up, the Senate had passed a measure reducing federal matching grants for optional services. It was later withdrawn, but its spirit informed the restraint on expansion of optional services in the years to come.

31. A number of the Great Society programs—for example, Model Cities and community mental health centers—bypassed state legislatures and forged a direct link between the federal government and localities, sometimes even neighborhoods.

32. One area of services where the federal government attempted even greater micromanagement was nursing home care, which was also the area of greatest expenditure in the Medicaid program. More than any other issue, this one tested the various divisions implicit in the original 1965 legislation. A fair proportion of the elderly overlapped the neat distinction between eligibility for health care as a right (under Medicare) and as a charity (under Medicaid). The expense of nursing home care frequently transferred the elderly from the first category to the second. Regulations increasingly attempted to specify the dividing line between health care and welfare and to clarify federal and state responsibilities (Vladeck 1980). Since Medicare was required to provide for nursing home care following a period of hospitalization, its provision could be considered as related to health care. To differentiate the skilled nursing home benefits under Medicaid from Medicare and health care, less stringent requirements for nursing home staff and facility standards were issued in 1967 (Sparer 1993). These Social Security amendments reflected federal concern for national safety standards primarily and established a federal role in monitoring minimal nursing home provisions. Whether responsibility for this function rested at the federal level, insofar as it had a significant fiscal if not ethical involvement, or with the states, in their capacity as licensing agencies, remained unclear for years, although the federal government tended to defer to the states. (The question is now coming to be settled as not an either-or issue but one that involves both levels of government.) Attempts to regulate the providers of nursing home care were further confused by their status as either administrators or entrepreneurs, but not necessarily professionals in either health or welfare. All of these distinctions, as well as the knots that tied them, became clearer as regulations increased, but at the same time the knots became tighter as loose ends began to appear.

33. In 1964 New York became the first state to require approval for capital expenditures by hospitals and nursing homes. By the time of the 1972 Social Security amendments sanctioning these developments, twenty-three states had followed suit with various conditions on facility construction, purchase of technology, and so on. The amendments empowered relevant government agencies to withhold or reduce Medicare and Medicaid reimbursement to hos-

pitals and nursing homes that were engaging in large capital expenditures not approved by state planning agencies.

34. The legislation specified only that approximately one-third of the membership be drawn from providers, government administrators, and for the first time, consumers.

35. However, those states with strong programs did hold down their costs to 3 percent below the national average. Campbell and Fournier (1993) suggest that the failure of states to contain hospital expenditures under the CON program may have been directly related to their success in achieving other goals. In particular, state governments were able to use their regulatory powers to promote subsidization of indigent care. Hackey (1993b:927) goes even further: Having achieved "other important policy objectives, such as increasing access to care for the uninsured and increasing lay participation in health policy planning, . . . state CON programs are poised to assume new roles during the 1990s."

36. New York began to switch from retrospective to prospective per diem rates in 1969, following an aborted attempt to impose a freeze on hospital rates. In 1971 New York became the first state to impose hospital rate regulation for Medicaid/Blue Cross reimbursement. The 1971 legislation contained too many exemptions, including countervailing wage increases, to be effective. Legislation in 1976 closed several loopholes and even closed some hospitals because of its new stringency. New legislation in 1978 reintroduced more liberal reimbursement within a context of revived interest-group politics. This legislation also established a state Council on Health Care Financing, which began work on an all-payer system in time for the politics of the 1980s (Hackey 1993a).

37. In some states the Blue Cross plans had set up semi-independent commissions to investigate bills and later to bargain over rates (Glaser 1984:706). As a result, commercial insurers became concerned about their competitiveness, especially with employers beginning to complain about the rising costs of insurance.

38. Also contained in section 1801 of the legislation was a section entitled "Prohibition Against Any Interference"; that is, by the federal government on providers. It became known as the "AMA clause" (Bjorkman 1989:50).

39. Physicians who participated were said to "accept assignment," meaning that they billed Medicare directly and accepted Medicare reimbursement in full. Nonparticipating physicians could bill their patients the full amount of their charges; these patients were then reimbursed by Medicare at a rate of 80 percent of the physicians' charge. In the case of nonparticipating physicians, Medicare acted like a standard indemnity insurance carrier, and Part B administration and provisions mirrored private insurance. Physicians were free to decide whether or not to participate on a case-by-case, claim-by-claim basis, thus continuing their ability to price-discriminate. Not until 1990 (OBRA 1989) were physicians required to accept assignment for patients whose copayments and deductions were covered by Medicaid. But physicians were not required to accept Medicaid patients (nor are they now), and many prefer not to. Continuing perhaps the legacy that health care for the poor ought to contain an element of charity, Medicaid has never fully reimbursed physicians for their services. However, some states might reimburse physicians more if their finances allowed. Over time, decreasing numbers of physicians have

accepted Medicaid patients, a negative exercise of their weakening power over health care financing.

40. In 1975 HEW sought to introduce more nonmedical personnel on the boards. Through the courts the AMA contested this overstepping of statutory authority, and won.

41. Programs in Maryland, Massachusetts, New Jersey, and New York are most commonly cited as the early successes (Ginsburg and Thorpe 1992:75). Hackey (1993a) notes the wide range of methods of control adopted by the more successful states; he calls these methods market-based (i.e., few state requirements), negotiated, and state-imposed.

42. The Social Security amendments of 1967 and 1972 authorized HEW to grant waivers for demonstration projects. In the 1970s federal agencies, not the states, generally initiated the few projects that qualified. Most of the early demonstrations focused on screening for children and home or community care for the frail or chronically ill. OBRA 1981 added a new category of programmatic waiver, which gave states more flexibility in developing innovations in the administration and delivery of Medicaid and which could be renewed indefinitely (unlike the time-limited demonstration waivers). The 1984 Deficit Reduction Act authorized waivers for HMO demonstration projects. Since 1965 approximately 80 so-called 1115 demonstration waivers have been granted, more than thirty of these since 1993; fifteen were pending as of early-1995 (Vladeck 1995:218). Waivers for HMO demonstrations are discussed in chapter 5.

43. Massachusetts, New York, and Maryland instituted what became known as all-payer hospital rate systems in the early 1980s; New Jersey, which was the site of the DRG demonstration project, applied the DRGs to all third-party payers.

44. The Prospective Payment Review Commission reported that inpatient hospital payments varied from approximately 80 percent of costs for the Medicaid program, 90 percent of costs for the Medicare program, and 128 percent of costs for private payers (Ginsburg and Thorpe 1992:76).

45. In 1991 Governor Weld (Republican) of Massachusetts excised the rate-setting commission and rescinded most of former Governor Dukakis' 1988 legislation for universal coverage, saving the 10 percent surtax on the bills of insured hospital patients to pay for the unemployed. California pioneered an alternative approach to hospital expenditure control under the Medicaid program that was initially attractive for emphasizing competition over regulation. Legislation in 1982 authorized state government actors to negotiate contracts with those hospitals that submitted the most cost-effective bids. Known as selective contracting, the approach carried additional features that bolstered its overall effect. Medi-Cal (the California Medicaid program) enrollees were restricted to care at hospitals with contracts. The definition of "medical necessity" was narrowed from services determined as necessary by the provider to services necessary "to protect life or prevent significant disability through the diagnosis or treatment of disease, illness or injury" (Preston et al. 1992:66). Hospitals without contracts could still provide emergency care and receive regular reimbursement. The "medically indigent adult" program (for low-income adults not meeting the categorical requirements for Medicaid) was eliminated

from Medi-Cal, and care of these individuals was transferred to the counties, with state funding support set at 70 percent of historical costs. Overall, then, competition was a small part of selective contracting. Officials at the state's negotiating commission acquired considerable power in actually "dictating" the prices hospitals could charge for Medi-Cal patients, eventually "snaring" a remarkable level of "centralized authority" (Sparer 1993:508). Within three years California's hospital expenditures under Medicaid were significantly reduced. Based on one-week samples taken before and after implementation, a HCFA study found that selective contracting resulted in a 23 percent saving over an estimate of costs if the program had not been implemented (Preston et al. 1992:66). The experiment paved the way for California to consider a state system of managed competition, which remains under discussion.

46. The DRG legislation instituted a system of prospective payment to hospitals under the Medicare program. It is based on approximately 470 categories of diseases or illnesses; the initial weightings were calculated as averages of past expenditures. The weightings are recalibrated periodically and include adjustments for the different experiences of urban/rural and teaching hospitals. Hospitals can keep any savings accrued, but if treatment exceeds the payment level, they are responsible for the difference. For the politics behind the development and passage of the DRG legislation, see Morone and Dunham (1985); for their social and political implications, see Ruggie (1992).

47. The PPRC, appointed in 1986, also provides independent expert advice to the secretary of HHS, especially regarding the calculations and updates of the fee scale. It is not an administrative body, however, and is not involved in implementation of the fee schedule. Nor does it work behind closed doors, as is HCFA's tendency, according to Oliver (1993).

48. The politics of developing the final version of the scale included disagreements between HCFA and PPRC. HCFA's recalculations resulted in greater decreases than the PPRC felt were acceptable to physicians, even though HCFA administrators claimed to have maintained close working relations with the profession's representatives. In the end Congress accepted the PPRC's higher calculations. It justified its recommendations, which were more receptive to physician concerns, with data on the following: growth in Part B expenditures, 70 percent of which went to physician payment; the "erratic" geographical variation in physician payment patterns (these figures were based on work by Wennberg; see, for example, Wennberg and Gittlesohn 1973); growth of physician incomes (in 1987 physician income in the United States was 4.8 times the income of an average full-time employee [PPRC 1989:25]); shifts in physician expenditure patterns since the introduction of the DRGs (e.g., more outpatient surgeries); and growth in out-of-pocket expenses by Medicare recipients.

49. The Medicare Fee Schedule is based on calculations of resource costs for average services (pre-, intra-, and postservices) within each specialty procedure in the Common Procedure Terminology, the standard nomenclature manual used by all physicians and third-party payers. Since the manual lists more than 7,000 procedures and some can be grouped (about 1,000 are for orthopedic surgery), not every procedure in a specialty was isolated. For the first phase of the study the researchers constructed a set of twenty to twenty-five scenarios of services commonly undertaken for each (grouped) procedure, and surveyed

about 185 practicing physicians in about 100 specialities. By 1992 values had been assigned for about 5,500 codes, adjusted for geographical differences in cost in about 230 localities. Among the items measured were amount of time, elements of intensity (physical effort and skill, mental effort and judgment, and stress), and practice costs. The PPRC changed the Hsiao team's measure of practice costs and, finding the measure of opportunity costs of advanced medical training to be redundant, eliminated it (PPRC 1989:31.).

50. Among the major recommendations of the PPRC was that refinement in coding evaluation and management services continue, since these tended to be undervalued relative to invasive procedures in the first phase of the study. Despite lobbying by surgeons, Congress rejected a separate schedule for surgical services and for certain other specialty groups that requested their own schedules. But Congress agreed to less harsh reductions in these fees and further study of the issues. Separate schedules were negotiated only for anesthesiologists and radiologists, and these are being phased in. As proposed by the PPRC, professional liability insurance has been extracted from other practice costs in calculating the values, and a new method of handling the complex issue of malpractice and its costs is under review.

51. PPRC (1995:399–408), which reports that almost 44 percent of Medicaid programs have adopted the Medicare Fee Schedule, as have approximately one-quarter of HMOs. Data are still not available on the adoption of the schedule by traditional fee-for-service insurers, but initial information is showing that some plans with billing and utilization restrictions are following Medicare's lead.

52. See note 39: Physicians who accepted assignment were formerly free to choose on a case-by-case, claim-by-claim basis.

53. It allowed participating physicians to charge 5 percent more than nonparticipating physicians on their deductible and copayment charges to patients; to continue to increase their charges despite a fee freeze in effect from 1984 to 1986 while nonparticipating physicians were required to obey the freeze; and to have their claims processed 7 days faster than nonparticipating physicians.

54. First, mandatory assignment for clinical laboratory services was required. OBRA 1986 created another restraint on physicians' extra-billing practices and in effect continued the fee freeze by setting a maximum allowable actual charge for nonparticipating physicians based on their 1984 charges. It also limited fee increases to 1 percent a year or up to a maximum of 115 percent of the "customary, prevailing, and reasonable" charge. In 1987 Congress began to specify more precisely annual increases in the Medicare Economic Index, as another tool to slow expenditure growth (PPRC 1992:12). By 1988, 77.3 percent of Medicare claims were on an assignment basis. The percentage of physicians who had signed Participating Physician and Supplier Program agreements (as a percentage of all physicians treating Medicare patients) remained at a steady 30 percent for the first few years of the program but jumped to 37.3 percent in the period from 1988 to 1989 (PPRC 1989:361). Physicians who have not signed Participating Physician and Supplier Program agreements can still choose assignment on a claim-by-claim basis. (See also Burney and Paradise [1987].)

55. It did not specify an amount (but presented simulations of limits ranging from 110 to 140 percent of the fee schedule).

56. Editorial, *American Medical News*, August 18, 1989, p. 1.

57. The PPRC first compared expenditure patterns in the United States, Canada, and Germany to support its case for volume controls. Its position was strengthened by data showing that in the United States growth in volume and intensity of services remained fairly steady throughout the 1980s but began to account for a larger proportion of expenditure in the late 1980s as controls on prices (the other main factor in expenditure increases) began to work (PPRC 1992:3–4; 1993:16). An equivalent form of volume control for specific factors within a global budget is missing in Canada. Introducing a VPS at this early stage of quasi-global budgeting in the United States may prevent the kind of turmoil in social relations that Canada has experienced.

58. Annual increases in the fee schedule are being phased in gradually at a rate of an additional 0.5 percent per year for the first few years (PPRC 1990:29). Its early consequences were therefore not radically different from what would have occurred under the Medicare Economic Index, which had previously determined fee increases.

59. When the Agency for Health Care Policy and Research first began developing practice guidelines, it focused its efforts on medical conditions (not treatments) in order to "dispel concern within the physician community that guidelines would be developed primarily as a cost containment tool. Having established its credibility, the agency may now be better positioned to address costs and cost-sensitive topics" (PPRC 1995:37).

Chapter Five

Privatization:
Blurred Boundaries or Beyond Boundaries?

Despite economic cycles of growth and retrenchment in their respective welfare states, government actors in Britain, Canada, and the United States have continued to adopt policies expanding public-sector provision of health care. In both Britain and Canada private-sector health care has taken a secondary role to public provision and has functioned to fill gaps left by the public sector. The opposite situation has prevailed in the United States, where public-sector measures have compensated for private-sector inequities or inadequacies. However, in all three countries, debates about the appropriateness of market forces shaping health care provision have intensified. Even in the United States, widespread concern has been voiced about the disparities in costs, profits, and services resulting from private enterprise. As a result, the role of the state in regulating health care has increased. The deficiencies of government's role in health care are still the target of considerable criticism in all three countries. But the fact that government is a fundamental actor in the field of health care is not an issue.

The previous three chapters presented the story of increasing state involvement in health care and suggested that state control

over private providers began to dissolve traditional liberal advoca-
cy of a separation between public and private rights and responsibilities. Welfare state development has proceeded on the widespread assumption that only the state can assure adequate, universal health care, and the state's role is therefore legitimate.
Nevertheless, in the 1980s governments undertook renewed attempts to control health care expenditures by introducing market
mechanisms to regulate supply and demand. Increasing constraints
accompanied economic recession. Chapter 1 argued that retrenchment in general has had mixed results, for although the state has
contained public expenditure growth and certain social programs
have suffered, overall expenditures have not been reduced. This
chapter demonstrates that the state has not pulled back from an
authoritative role in guiding a broader social base of health care
provision.

The consequences of retrenchment become even more complex
when we explore its flip side, privatization. The reappearance of
privatization in the 1980s raised familiar questions about public-
sector accountability.[1] For instance, if state divestiture is occurring, what is happening to the state's responsibility for the needy?
Moreover, is the state actively encouraging an increase in the role
of the private sector in welfare state programs—and if so, what kind
and how much? Above all, what are the consequences of private-
sector provision for equity and justice in health care?

The answers that were given throughout the 1980s invoked the
principles and norms of separate roles and relations. A shift from
public to private-sector responsibility for social provision was justified as relieving the state of burdens it could no longer shoulder.
A rollback in state provision was further justified by failures in the
achievements of government intervention, which had not produced
the efficiency and effectiveness in health care that had been expected. In Britain, Canada, and the United States, economic uncertainties supported increasing separation between public and private,
state and market, regulation and competition. Market-based or private-sector efforts were expected to replace the supposedly failed
mechanisms of state intervention with opposing and supposedly
more vibrant modes of organizing health care. But the consequences have turned out to be different from what was expected.

Privatization in contemporary liberal welfare states is a multifaceted and complicated phenomenon. To understand its complex-

ity, let us turn first to definitions. Several empirically different definitions are tied by a common conceptual embeddedness in the classical liberal paradigm of a segmentation in the domains of state and society. Lundqvist (1988:1), for instance, proposes that privatization "is the active and conscious transfer of responsibility from the public to the private realm," involving three main activities: regulation, financing, and production. Starr (1989:22).also proposes a definition of privatization as a shift in the production of goods and services. But he wants to leave "open the possibility that privatization may not actually result in less government spending and regulation—indeed, may unexpectedly increase them." Be that as it may, Starr cannot overcome his fundamental "distrust" of privatization and "fear" of its power-base among conservatives (1989:44). Kamerman (1989:262) supports Starr's distrust by dismissing the efficiency–economy–choice arguments for privatization, claiming they are not proven by the evidence. She concludes that privatization can only be supported by an ideological stance against government.

Some studies of privatization attempt to avoid zero-sum analysis of separate spheres by describing ambiguous intersections between public and private domains. For instance, Smith and Stone (1988:242) find that the

> privatization strategy of contracting for social services with private nonprofit agencies has not involved a simple devolution of programs from the public sector to the private sector, as though one were handing the baton to the other, but rather a penetration of the state into the private sector. This penetration has in some ways strengthened the private welfare system (by giving it public funds, expanding it, and mobilizing it as a political constituent) and in some ways weakened it (by encumbering it with all the red tape of public bureaucracy and by rendering it dependent on the vagaries of public funding).

This chapter adopts a similar argument. It maintains that conceptual dichotomies between public and private, state and market, regulation and competition are inadequate to understand fully current developments in health care provision. It suggests that contemporary relations between any set of conceptually dichotomous spheres are best understood as interfused. For instance, the state has adopted certain market-based processes, such as competition in public programs, at the same time that it is attempting to deter market forces from eroding equality in access and provision. For their part, some private-sector providers seem to have incorporated public-sector goals, limiting their profit-maximizing objectives in order to achieve a more equitable distribution of resources. For example, troubled as the U.S. Medicaid program may be, provider acquiescence to its presence, including private absorption of unpaid costs, indicates a measure of acceptance of responsibility for social provision. To understand these activities, we can refer to the policy regimes framework. The new roles and relations between public- and private-sector actors are not well captured by the terms of a segmented policy regime, because a separation of domains no longer pertains. Nor are the terms of an interventionist policy regime appropriate, because of the greater give and take that seems to be occurring between the two sectors. To the extent that we can focus on this give and take, the intermingling of roles, and the social construction of new relations, we can turn to the terms of an integrative policy regime.

The main argument of this book is that the welfare state is not being dismantled, although the role of the state is changing. Moreover, current changes in the role of the state may represent not attrition but potential enhancement of state capacity. Chapter 1 argued that whether or not retrenchment includes an actual reduction of state provision, it does involve a shift in the role of the state from ever-increasing public provision to greater authoritative oversight of broader-based social provision. So too may privatization represent an increase in the role of the private sector for the broader public purpose of providing health care within terms mutually constructed with state actors. In other words, there is a form of privatization that results in the state being more able to guide the private sector toward collective purposes. That form of privatization is the focus of this chapter.

In all three countries during the 1980s conservative governments adopted privatization measures and justified these as offering economic and political improvements over state-centered provision. Although some shift from public to private ownership, production, financing, delivery, or regulation occurred in the provision of various social services, in none of the three countries has the responsibility of the state declined as a result. A "return" of health care to private auspices has not occurred. Instead, we can say that the contribution of both public and private sectors for this particular welfare state program has increased. The instances of privatization in British, Canadian, and American health care examined in the following sections have been selected to demonstrate different empirical formats within a similar, emergent, structural form.

Britain

The private sector (for-profit and nonprofit) has always been a presence in British health care. Before the 1980s the roles and relations of public- and private-sector actors were generally contained within the institutional framework characteristic of a segmented policy regime. There was minimal public regulation of private activities. Harley Street, famous for its prestigious physicians who perform most of their services in private facilities, has long been an enclave of essentially untouched privilege.[2] Links between private-practice physicians and the public sector have occurred indirectly, insofar as most consultants also work for the NHS. How they carry public-sector rules over to their private practices is up to them. Private-sector health care in Britain has been the mainstay for those activities the NHS has explicitly chosen not to fund, such as fertilization procedures and sterilization as a method of birth control.[3] Since 1980, increasingly more elective surgeries have also been performed in the private sector, for those who have supplementary private insurance or can otherwise afford to "jump the queue." Despite the presence and recent growth of private health care in Britain, its overall size remains small compared to the public sector, whether measured as a percentage of total expenditures or size of budget or level of activity.[4] Even if the private sector continues to grow, it is expected to account for no more than 20 percent of total health care in Britain. Numbers notwithstanding, the contribution of private health care has been significant; but it has not damaged the NHS.

The early years of the Thatcher administration witnessed an unprecedented growth in private-sector health care.[5] Thatcher's initiatives had several objectives. Many scholars agree that the professed goal of obtaining more "value for money" was superseded by the not-so-hidden agenda of restructuring government by limiting its reach and replacing the public sector with private provision (Krieger 1986; Brush 1987). The Thatcher government attempted to

impose an actual shift from public to private ownership and production in health care by selling off some hospitals and facilities.[6]
Their loss was not altogether shattering because many were older
facilities and expensive to keep. Most of the increase in the private
sector during the 1980s was due not to a shift, but to actual private-
sector growth. More important, it did not involve an absolute
decline in public-sector activity.

The consequences of an increase in the role of the private sector
are subject to many interpretations. I contend that diminishing the
supremacy of the NHS is not among them, even though the NHS has
been relieved of its overload. To demonstrate the nature of privatization in British health care, I briefly examine three areas where it
has been most prominent: insurance, user fees, and contracting.
What is most significant is that the emerging roles of public and
private actors in Britain are unlike those in earlier eras, when the
state either adopted a hands-off approach to the private sector or
attempted to shape private behavior through intrusive regulations.
Instead, various efforts at mutual accommodation are suggestive of
an integrative policy regime.

Private Insurance

An early initiative of the Thatcher government was to propose that
incentives be provided for British citizens to buy private insurance.
Although the proposal did not advance much beyond rhetoric, private insurance attracted many new subscribers during the early
1980s.[7] Whether because no explicit incentives to buy private
insurance had materialized by 1985, save the threat of dismantling
parts of the NHS, or because premiums rose (95 percent in real terms
over the course of the 1980s), the rate of growth in new subscriptions dropped in the mid- to late 1980s. Nevertheless, by the late
1980s more than 3 million people, constituting more than 10 percent of the population, carried some form of private insurance.

In an effort to regenerate interest in private insurance, the 1989
White Paper, *Working for Patients*, proposed income tax relief on
premiums purchased by persons over the age of 60 and individuals
earning less than £8,500 per year. This tax relief provided insufficient incentive to increase the subscription rate of the elderly or
lower-income groups. Moreover, as a mechanism to increase private purchases of health insurance, the proposal overlooked the

main population of buyers. Private insurance coverage is concentrated among middle-aged members of the more affluent socioeconomic groups living in and around London.[8] In addition, many new policies are purchased by companies as part of an employee benefits package.[9] By the early 1990s, company purchase began to decline whereas individual and group purchases continued to increase, albeit more slowly. Still, approximately three-quarters of private insurance subscriptions are held through employers.[10]

The overall impact of private insurance on health care in general and the NHS in particular has been modest. Benefits offered by most private insurance policies are limited and carry typical restrictions (for instance, most preexisting conditions are not covered, outpatient visits are not covered in some plans, and there are limits on reimbursement). Pregnancy is the only procedure explicitly excluded in British private insurance (only 1 percent of babies in Britain are born outside of the NHS). Table 5.1 indicates that private insurance tends to be used more for hospital amenities (including private beds in NHS hospitals) than for the services of specialists. Provision for screening procedures (fitness assessment; special examinations for women, men, or the elderly; and so on) grew throughout the 1980s, outstripping screening procedures offered within the NHS. Screening for specific kinds of cancer is increasing in the NHS, but at a slow pace, providing the private sector with a potential growth area. The NHS applies fairly restrictive age-based rules of eligibility for initial and follow-up screenings, which also opens the market for private-sector uptake (Laing and Buisson 1988/89:36). However, screening is only a preparatory health care service and a means to another end. When test results are used by NHS doctors, an interpenetration of spheres occurs.

TABLE 5.1 *Private Insurance Benefits—Britain*

TYPE OF MEDICAL CARE	1977	1988
Room charges	50.2%	44.0%
Surgeons and anesthetists' fees	23.3	22.5
Inpatient physicians' and specialists' fees	4.4	3.5
Outpatient specialists' fees	15.2	14.8
Miscellaneous inpatient and outpatient fees	6.9	15.1
	100%	100%

Source: Adapted from Laing and Buisson (1992:43).

Thus, the use of private insurance reflects the features of a segmented policy regime on the surface only. There are many points of intersection, indeed interdependence, between the public and private sectors, suggesting that elements of an integrative framework have evolved.

The Thatcher government attempted to make private insurance more central to health care by halting the closure of pay beds in NHS hospitals and by removing certain restrictions on private hospital development.[11] Several American corporations—such as American Medical International, Humana, and the Hospital Corporation of America—responded by setting up branches of their hospital chains, mostly with specialized services in newly constructed buildings. Within a decade the number of beds in American for-profit hospitals exceeded that in other private-sector facilities save charity hospitals (Laing and Buisson 1988/89:24–27). By the late 1980s, however, an oversupply of beds led to sellouts. At present the private hospital sector is dominated by two British companies and one American (American Medical International). About 56 percent of private beds are for-profit (up from 29 percent in 1979); the remainder are in religious or charitable nonprofit hospitals (Calnan, Cant, Gabe 1993:5).

This growth in private hospital beds went hand in hand with an increase in private-sector surgeries. By 1986 a visible change appeared in the proportion of elective surgeries being performed in the private sector, as Table 5.2 demonstrates. It should be emphasized that elective surgeries, not emergencies, were most affected. It is possible, then, that one consequence of privatization might be a reduction in waiting lists for elective surgeries. Data are beginning to show some successes in certain districts in reducing the number of people on NHS waiting lists, especially those who have

TABLE 5.2 *Surgeries—Britain*

INPATIENT ELECTIVE SURGERIES	1981		1986	
	CASES	%	CASES	%
Independent hospitals*	162,100	9.8	286,700	14.9
NHS pay beds	57,500	3.5	35,700	1.9
NHS remainder	1,440,900	86.8	1,603,900	83.8
All sectors	1,660,500	100.0	1,926,300	100.0

*Excluding NHS patients treated in independent hospitals under contractual arrangements.

Source: Adapted from Laing and Buisson (1988/89:12).

been waiting for more than a year (Laing and Buisson 1993:136–37). But further analysis is needed to determine the extent to which privatization is the cause.

Other data on the public/private mix of selected services indicate that the majority of health care remains under the NHS (Laing and Buisson 1988–1989:5; 1992:63). Moreover, the government maintains a modicum of regulatory power over all non-NHS facilities. It can be expected to increase as local health authorities use private facilities more under the evolving contractual arrangements discussed later.

In sum, although these uses of private insurance have increased private-sector provision of health care, they do not pose a threat to the stability of the NHS. Private-sector insurance is best considered as an adjunct or complement to the NHS. It is used less for essential services and benefits than for those that are in short supply in the NHS, providing care for patients on long elective surgery queues and fulfilling excess demand for amenities. Individuals with private insurance continue to use the NHS for an estimated four-fifths of their outpatient appointments and one-half of their in-patient stays (Day and Klein 1989). In some areas of provision, private insurance offers alternative funding for services that are integral to health care (such as tests that NHS doctors can utilize). This interfacing of spheres of responsibility is new in the NHS in this area of insurance. Its introduction at this time is beginning to substantiate the framework of an integrative policy regime.

User Fees

Privatization has also occurred within the NHS itself. One form is commodification of formerly "free" items. For instance, the NHS has expanded the use of private copayments for prescriptions.[12] Also, in 1985 the government began to exclude certain medicines (mainly common remedies for nonserious ailments) from NHS reimbursement. However, because of exemptions (for example, for pregnant women, the elderly, low income families, and people suffering from certain disabilities), 82 percent of all prescriptions dispensed in Britain remain free of charge. Despite a decline in its purchasing power, the NHS continues as a monopsony buyer of privately produced pharmaceuticals, with 63 percent of the market. Charges for dental care have also increased. Eyeglasses are no longer covered by the NHS except for children, low-income groups, and those with complex vision needs. These various increases in private payments contribute a mere 3 percent to the NHS coffers.

Commodification is also evident in the increasing number of pay beds in public hospitals.[13] Although some of the larger teaching hospitals in London have converted entire wings to privately paid provision, the proportion of private beds in any single NHS hospital remains small. Indeed, it is expected to decline, because the venture has not been profitable. Less than one-third of pay beds are in use on any one day, and although they account for almost one-quarter of all private beds in Britain, they generate only one-tenth of the revenue (Laing and Buisson 1988–1989:16).[14] The NHS could improve its pricing system to be more in line with private-sector charges; most local authorities seem to be opting instead for alternative methods of enhancing competitiveness.

Contractual Arrangements

A similarly ambiguous fate has accompanied the experiment with contracting out as a form of privatization in the NHS. A Local Government Planning and Land Act, passed in 1980, first required that the public sector compete with the private market for all work valued above a certain amount per job. Follow-up circulars from the Department of Health and Social Services (DHSS) modified this directive and applied it to the NHS, suggesting that local health authorities solicit bids for "domestic and laundry services, maintenance of buildings and vehicles, security services and transport services . . . catering, computers, any pharmaceutical or other manufacturing for which there is an alternative commercial supply, and indeed any other services where you may see scope."[15]

Very little contracting out actually occurred during the 1980s. While all local authorities endeavored to procure bids, several found the results in savings not worth the effort. In addition, the new administrative tasks of comparing bids, drafting contracts, monitoring standards, and channeling patients confronted local authorities with legal responsibilities for which they were unprepared and to which they were unwilling to devote yet more resources (Chandra and Kakabadse 1985:57).

Contractual arrangements are at the heart of management changes in the new self-governing hospital trusts and in independent fundholding by GPs and local health authorities, as discussed in chapter 2. Under these initiatives, purchasers of health care are free to develop their own terms with whichever providers they chose. Nevertheless, freedom is constrained by the expenditure caps of global budgeting. The regulations that do exist induce competition for the best price, a process the British refer to as "managed competition" (King's Fund 1989). It entails the same concerns about underservicing as exist in the United States. Assuagement of both the concern and the possible underservicing will require enhancement and enforcement of quality assurance programs.

Labor Resources

Although contracting out is a significant form of privatization in and of itself, it was more important at first for the opportunity it afforded the government to force a wedge into union power. Conservatives had long held that wasteful employment practices had been allowed to permeate the NHS, as in other strongly unionized public-sector industries, damaging public-sector adaptability and efficiency. As with all health care systems, labor costs in the NHS are a large part of the budget, which makes them a prime target for reductions. The Thatcher attack on NHS labor reflected her administration's ideology (Pulkingham 1989). On the assumption that labor should compete in the marketplace like any other commodity, the central government abolished the fair wages clause (Mohan and Woods 1985:199). Unionized workers were put in the situation of having to compete with nonunionized (and lower-paid) workers in their contracting bids. Local authorities, who do some hiring on their own, acted cautiously, wondering if the central government recognized the "major industrial relations problems" entailed by its actions (Chandra and Kakabadse 1985:63). The success of this attempt at opening the NHS to market forces was minimal. By the 1990s the hold of collective bargaining in determining the wages of unionized employees had not decreased, and nonunionized, lower-paid workers had not been hired en masse. Even though self-governing hospital trusts now have the right to negotiate their own labor contracts, they also remain mindful of past agreements with unions.

Nurses have been particularly affected by privatization. The employment of nurses in the private sector has increased substantially. In fact, there is a concern that private-sector employment may be stealing nurses from the public sector. In 1985 the private sector employed 7 percent of the total nursing workforce, and 42 percent came directly from the NHS (Propper 1989:6–7). Nevertheless, the private sector remains dependent on the public sector for nurse training, which could be interpreted either as interlinking of sectors or as syphoning.

More than any other labor resource, physicians could be most affected by the surge of possibilities for privatization in health care. In 1980 the NHS formed a new contract with hospital consultants, allowing those working full-time for the NHS to engage in limited private practice, not to exceed 10 percent of their gross income. At present approximately 50 percent of NHS consultants have such full-time contracts. About 35 percent of NHS consultants have maximum part-time contracts, which allow them to undertake unlimited private practice in return for foregoing one-eleventh of their NHS salaries. The remaining consultants have various pro-rated, part-time contracts. It is estimated that approximately 100 specialists in Britain do not have contracts with the NHS, compared to 15,000 with full- and part-time contracts. Thus, some NHS patients in Britain are being cared for by the same physicians who care for private patients. At the same time, because of part-time contracts for specialists, the private outpatient sector within the NHS is growing. Its success rests, however, on the ability of private insurance and private hospitals to accommodate demand, limited though that demand may be.

Conclusion

The thrust of these developments in privatization in Britain can be summarized as aimed at behavioral changes stemming from fuller awareness among providers and purchasers of the costs of health care. The stated goal is improved efficiency; although it was assumed that expenditure reduction would result, it has not. In the late 1980s overall health expenditure dipped below 6 percent of GDP in Britain. By the early 1990s it was rising more than ever (see chapter 6, table 6.2). Privatization did uncover inefficiencies in the NHS and guided corrective measures. However, the consequences of privatization on effectiveness in overall provision of health care have not yet been investigated. It also remains to be seen to what extent the NHS will practice what it requires of others and plow savings back into health care in order to enhance quality. Some of this might already be occurring, given recent expenditure data. Nevertheless, privatization has reinforced the central role of government as chief overseer of a broader social base of provision. The form that government regulation now takes is not well described as intrusion, nor is government assuming a hands-off attitude toward private-sector activities (recall its regulation of private insurance, the exemptions for prescription payments, etc.). Both of these stances were characteristic of earlier policy regimes. If the mutually adjustive roles that have been described here continue and enable the construction of a relationship geared toward common goals in health care provision and outcome, it will suggest the emergence of an integrative policy regime tying the public and private sectors together in an overall system of health care.

Canada

The private portion of overall health care expenditure in Canada is about 25 percent, and its domain is limited by law to those benefits and services not provided by the public program. The law therefore affirms separate spheres of rights and responsibilities. However, practice has broken down traditional barriers, enabling more accommodative roles and relationships between public and private-sector actors.

Take, for instance, the jurisdictional locations of health care providers, beginning with hospitals. Privatization as ownership is minimal in Canadian hospitals. There are a few for-profit specialty hospitals and nursing homes (3 percent of total), but their numbers are not growing because they are strictly regulated by law. By and large, then, hospital ownership is public or voluntary. Privatization in regulatory control of hospitals is more prevalent but still ambiguous. The governance of hospitals is decentralized and "private" in that all hospitals are headed by lay boards of trustees. Among other functions, these boards decide whether a hospital should raise its own revenues for capital projects. However, provincial government approval is required for all capital projects; in addition, all other hospital operating costs are negotiated through global budgeting.

Turning next to physicians, we can say that similar forms of segmentation and regulation describe in the abstract the roles and relations of government actors and physicians. Although all physicians own their private practices, all are reimbursed through the provincial insurance system. In principle, physicians can opt out of the insurance system, but because in most provinces opted-out physicians are not reimbursed by public insurance, very few do. In Ontario opted-out physicians cannot charge more than the plan's reimbursement level. It is this combination of public governance and private ownership (physicians) and private governance and public ownership (hospitals) that underpins current and evolving movement toward privatization in Canada.

Unlike Britain and the United States, Canada was not governed in the 1980s by ideological advocates of increased privatization in health care.[16] Nevertheless, the role of the private sector and its contribution to overall health care expenditure did increase, all at the provincial level because of the shift away from federal financing that followed the 1977 Established Programs Financing Act. To the extent that privatization is contained within the framework of public regulation and to the extent that all providers understand that the intent of that framework is to provide equitable, basic health care, privatization has rendered little substantial change in Canada's health care system. Within this regulatory framework mechanisms that in the United States are touted as cost containment, such as coinsurance, are recognized in Canada as expanding overall expenditure on health care (Weller and Manga 1983:501). Private-sector contributions allow the public-sector portion to be contained but not necessarily reduced. A question that remains of concern, however, is how far privatization will go and with what consequences for universal and comprehensive health care. Can Canadians be assured that the basic tenets of public insurance embodied in the Canada Health Act—equality in access above all— will remain intact? Since the Canada Health Act does not specify the substance of basic health care, will deterioration occur? I briefly examine three main areas of privatization in Canada—supplementary insurance, nursing home care, and hospital management—to elucidate the limits of the privatization ventures underway and to explore the applicability of the model of an integrative policy regime.

Supplementary Private Insurance

The role of private health insurance in Canada decreased considerably with the passage of Medicare, but it did not die out.[17] Although the public insurance system is comprehensive, it is not complete. For instance, dental care and ambulatory prescription drugs are not covered under the national legislation or by any provincial program. Besides providing coverage for noninsured services, private insurance is available for private or semiprivate hospital rooms, medical devices (eyeglasses, hearing aids, wheelchairs), and diagnostic tests performed in private laboratories. Supplementary insurance is also available for short- and long-term disability and for those traveling outside of Canada (especially important for emergency treatment of visitors in the United States). Table 5.3 summarizes the number of people who carry private coverage for various benefits. Most of the purchasers are employers; in most private plans individuals are responsible for some premium and copayment contributions. In general terms the relationships between public- and private-sector insurance are similar in Canada and Britain. But because there is more private insurance in Canada, its implications for access to and comprehensiveness of health care are more momentous.

The separate roles of actors in the public and private insurance systems in Canada evoke the characteristics of a segmented policy

TABLE 5.3 *Private Insurance Benefits—Canada**

	ESTIMATED NUMBERS COVERED[†]		
	TOTAL	INSURED PLANS		UNINSURED[††] PLANS
	1990	1980	1990	1990
Extended health care	17,687	10,081	12,437	5,250
Supplementary hospital only	na	na	1,899	na
Dental	11,556	5,876	6,970	4,586

*Data are for companies doing 97% of the business.
[†]Thousands.
[††]Employers' benefits outside insurance contract, not guaranteed by insurance company.

Source: Adapted from CLHIA *(1991:46–47).*

regime. Indeed, industry representatives recognize that "Private insurance takes off where government coverage ends" (CLHIA 1991:44). However, although both the amount of government regulation and the opportunities for expansion in private insurance are circumscribed, a more fluid boundary appears to be emerging between the two domains as supplementary private insurance grows. Continuing fluidity rests on government's willingness to base its future decisions to contain public insurance on the capacity of the private sector to fill any gaps that arise. There is considerable concern in Canada about the consequences of additional government "deinsurance" of certain benefits. To contain expenditures, some provinces have eliminated previously covered services. Some of these cuts have been justified by substantive norms differentiating "essential" versus "nonessential" services. For example, Alberta has ceased to cover any cosmetic surgery. Other cuts are more difficult to justify. Physical therapy provision, which already varies among provincial plans, seems particularly vulnerable to further cuts. The same is true for mental health care, which many provinces limit by specifying the number and kinds of reimbursable services. Government actors seem to be testing the capacity of the market to absorb government retrenchment. As long as this continues, privatization of supplementary insurance will constitute a transfer from public- to private-sector responsibility, and a reinforcement of separate spheres in terms of market rationality. However, if the public and private sectors were to collaborate more before experimenting with changes in coverage—for instance, by negotiating reasonable payments and provider mechanisms to maintain necessary and optimum levels of care—a more integrative policy regime could begin to take hold.

Nursing Home Care

More than any other area of health care provision, long-term care for the elderly in Canada suggests the emergence of an integrative policy regime. Nursing home care is undergoing significant change, and developments in privatization are shedding past layers of segmented roles and relations. Provincial governments are not encouraging an increase in the role of the private sector so much as a change in the type of provision: from institutional to home care. The overall contribution of the private sector to elder care may increase as a result, but in its new form it will be under greater government regulation. Already proprietary nursing home operators complain that government regulations encumber them more than comparable regulation of public-sector facilities, a reflection perhaps of a somewhat suspicious attitude on the part of Canadian government officials toward for-profit motives (Fried, Deber, Leatt 1987:577). Although the complaints imply government intrusion into private affairs, they could also constitute the first steps in an interlinking of sectors that could pave the way for mutually supportive roles and collaborative relations. Although a mix of policy regimes exists at present, because developments are new, some sorting out can be expected. The direction depends, of course, on the degree to which roles and relations are divisible.

The specifics of nursing home care vary by province; Ontario illustrates well the character of change. Ontario is among the more politically conservative provinces in Canada, making it a favorable locale for all aspects of privatization. In the past, long-term care for the elderly reflected the great public/private divide characteristic of a segmented policy regime. The proportion of specialty long-term care beds for the elderly in for-profit facilities has always outnumbered provision in public or charitable facilities.[18] Yet the first provincial regulations of for-profit facilities did not appear until 1966, and not until 1972 was funding assistance available. For twenty years provincial financial assistance for care in proprietary facilities remained lower than for comparable care provided by public and charitable facilities. Private providers complained about the lack of support and used it to excuse recriminations against them for inadequacies in care.[19] Moreover, Ontario remained the only province to perpetuate the legacy of divided governmental jurisdictions between public and private facilities for long-term care for the elderly and the accompanying stigma of welfare for the elderly poor—the Ministry of Health regulated private nursing homes, and the Ministry of Community and Social Service governed public and charitable facilities. These past circumstances make the current changes all the more meaningful.

Beginning with a Liberal provincial administration in the 1980s and continuing with the New Democratic Party in the 1990s, provincial governments have been attempting to reduce and perhaps eliminate the differences between public and private long-term care for the elderly. Three main mechanisms work in tandem. First, all facilities and related services for the elderly are gradually being brought under the administrative framework of a new, unified Division of Community Health and Support Services/Long Term Care Branch in the provincial government. Division administrators are attempting to standardize quality, inspection, and accreditation criteria, pending further legislation.

Second, the financing structure of facilities and related services is gradually being rationalized, in terms of both the fiduciary role of the provincial government and the structure of user fees. In the past, per diem fees for private nursing home patients were negotiated annually between the Ministry of Health and the Ontario Nursing Home Association, a process that resulted in separate and lower subsidization rates for certain patients in private facilities compared with those in public or charitable facilities. In contrast, funding for public and charitable facilities was conducted through global budgeting, which offered these facilities more flexibility in distributing their resources according to different levels of patient care needs. At the same time, user fees varied among facilities; the extent of this discrepancy was unknown because private facilities kept their books closed. In the 1970s the provincial government began to intervene through legislation requiring full disclosure of the terms of patients' payments (semi/private rooms, hours of nursing care, etc.). Different fee structures still remain within and among facilities, but facilities are now legally accountable for the differences. In addition, standardization in residential fees among the facilities is occurring; for example, there is now a fixed copayment for extended care regardless of facility,[20] and every patient must be able to retain a minimum of approximately $115 (Cdn) per month (adjusted annually for cost of living increases) as a "comfort" or personal spending allowance. Nonliquid assets are no longer taken into account in determining ability to pay; however, patients with liquid assets are steered away from public assistance. Ultimately, decisions about level of care are made by doctors; facility placement decisions are up to social workers. The Ontario Health Insurance Program pays all medical costs and whatever nursing home fee remains after patient payments are met.

A third assault on the public/private divide in elder care is occurring through reconceptualization of appropriate types of accommodation for varying needs. Although every elderly Canadian has the right to long-term care in a public facility if needed, medically and financially, the provincial government in Ontario is attempting to redefine levels of need and to encourage home or community-based care in lieu of institutional care where appropriate or possible. Limits have been placed on the expansion of institutional beds in public facilities, but the private sector remains free to accommodate market demand as it judges best. Placement of government-subsidized elderly (that is, the poor) in private facilities is already increasing, though on a small scale. The private sector is expanding in the new market for home-based care, and the provincial government is developing contractual arrangements for such services on a case-management basis. A wide variety of services is available as a right, subject to physician determination of need.[21] Contractual arrangements with private providers will most likely outpace public-sector provision of the many services that constitute home and community-based care.

In sum, because public facilities are rapidly moving away from institutional care, the private sector is temporarily filling a gap. Although private nursing home care is not increasing, intermediate care is expanding. Analytically speaking, in their roles and relations public- and private-sector actors show a new flexibility and willingness to collaborate. Whether in deciding on the amount an individual should contribute toward his/her long-term care or in deciding on the type of home care or facility needed, former boundaries between public and private rights and responsibilities are in principle being ignored in favor of solving the problem of care for the elderly. Relations between public and private sectors are coming to be based more on contractual arrangements, which specify the terms of payment and provision. Although there is no government regulation of noncontractual elements, such as the abstract obligation to provide quality services, oversight is now more widespread.

Hospital Management

The largest institutional component of health care—hospitals—is also the most expensive. Most hospitals in Canada are publicly owned (more than 75 percent of approved beds are in public general hospitals), most of the remainder are voluntary facilities, and a small proportion (about 3 percent) are proprietary. In addition, hospital expenditures constitute a greater proportion of overall health care expenditures in Canada than in Britain or the United States (see chapter 6, figure 6.6). It might be expected, then, that any movement toward privatization would affect hospitals more than any other area. Privatization in the hospital sector has not taken the form of a shift in ownership; instead it has focused on management. Specifically, hospitals have contracted with private firms to manage their provision of care.

There is a fairly clear distinction in Canada between hospital administration, governance, and management. By law, health care is publicly administered, which means that the terms of public provision cannot be implemented by private insurance companies. All hospitals are governed by boards of trustees, who are for the most part community members (physicians are not board members but can participate in discussions; some hospitals have placed nurses on board committees) (Baker 1992). The management of hospitals—that is, the day-to-day implementation of policies—is by and large conducted "in-house" by salaried executives. However, a few hospitals in Canada have endeavored to achieve greater cost control by turning to private-sector management firms—for inspiration if not actual assistance.

Ontario has developed a hybrid form of privatization in management, relying on the power of incentives contained in private-sector management techniques. In 1982 the provincial government initiated a Business Oriented New Development program, whereby hospitals were encouraged to consolidate accounting and meet all their expenditures from existing budgets, a more thorough form of global budgeting than before (Fried, Deber, Leatt 1987:578). The main innovation was permitting hospitals to keep any savings that resulted and holding them responsible for their own deficits.[22] Some of the methods of cost control identified by the Ministry of Health and adopted by hospitals included multiunit management, sharing of services among units, and contracting out for services. In a spillover effect, multihospital arrangements for the management and purchase of materials and services also began, in Ontario as well as in a number of other provinces. Eventually, some hospital mergers occurred too.

These initiatives in hospital management are more correctly referred to as corporatization and not privatization, insofar as they represent the adoption of a specific organizational form "characterized by clearly articulated corporate objectives and a division between corporate and operational levels" (Fried, Deber, Leatt 1987:568). However, four cases of actual privatization of hospital management have occurred in Canada, in which for-profit firms have been retained to manage service delivery and accounting procedures in hospitals (or in one case a large hospital wing). In one hospital in Ontario, American Medical International, which received an annual fee for a twelve-year contract, eliminated the deficit, achieved a surplus, and introduced improvements in a number of functions, including staff education and communication between the hospital's board and administrative staff (Stoddart and Labelle 1985:19–21). As studies elaborate the best methods of achieving savings, it may not be necessary to hire private firms to improve hospital efficiencies—arguably, to be sure.

Whether or not these initiatives are the cause, recent studies show more favorable figures for overall hospital productivity. There has been an overall decline in the number of hospitals in Canada, yielding a higher bed occupancy rate.[23] In addition, low inpatient service productivity figures are apparently being offset by improvements in productivity for outpatient services.[24]

Conclusion

The hold of segmented roles and relations is strong in Canada. Although developments in privatization portend possible reversion to the bifurcated roots of health care provision, overall the trend toward increasing private-sector responsibility is being held in check by Canada's commitment to a public program of universal and comprehensive health insurance coverage. Private-sector adherence to the governing rules of this program does not require strong intervention on the part of government actors. But some regulation and legislation do structure and oversee the responsibilities of private-sector actors. Privatization in Canada has taken a number of different forms. It functions as an adjunct to the public program in the case of supplementary insurance. In other areas, however, particularly long-term care for the elderly, public- and private-sector provision appears to be integrated within an overall framework of care for the elderly. Representatives from the two sectors negotiate the terms of care on a case-by-case basis. This experimentation with privatization not only leaves Canada's national program undamaged, but also goes further in enhancing the capacity of the nation to extend the meaning of fundamental rights to care.

The United States

There was considerable debate in the 1980s about whether health care provision and delivery would be subject to a choice between regulation or competition. On the surface the choice seemed moot. Increasing government intervention in what has always been predominantly private-sector health care had clearly failed to control costs. By the early 1980s the conservative agenda of returning to market forces seemed to emerge victorious. It was unclear, though, exactly how the market worked in health care, let alone if the market and the competition it wrought were even appropriate in this area of social provision.[25] Thus, much sorting out persisted during the 1980s. The entrenched boundaries between public versus private, regulation versus competition, state versus market were open to debate once again. In the end, the responsibilities of *both* the government and the private sector in health care were reaffirmed.

Although private provision of health care is growing in the United States, the private sector is also engaging in a novel form of self-regulation that involves the incorporation of rules and standards set by the government. At the same time, government actors are adopting market-based incentives in public-sector provision of health care. This interweaving of organizing principles and norms is not a confusing mix of policy regimes. It contains a unique pragmatism that did not occur in the past.

Recent developments have not involved an actual shift from public to private health care in the United States, nor is privatization taking the form of cooptation of the private sector for public purposes.[26] However, government regulation and legislation pertaining to private-sector provision of health care have grown. If this alone were occurring, the discussion could not go much beyond an analysis of the evolution from a segmented to an interventionist policy regime. The following presentation suggests that more may be occurring. Public- and private-sector actors in the United States seem to be engaged in constructing a common understanding of what constitutes adequate care. Both sets of actors are modifying past practices, and in so doing they are making way for a common standard of care. These newly emerging roles and relations are suggestive of an integrative policy regime.

I have chosen to illustrate these possibilities through an examination of HMOs because of the central role they have come to play in American health care policy.[27] An evolution in policy regimes is discernible in the principles that have governed HMOs. The increasingly more collaborative decision making that occurs between HMO representatives and government actors offers a model of innovation in health care.

HMOs: Evolution in Public/Private Relations

From their origins as grassroots, self-help, cooperative movements in the Depression era, prepaid group insurance plans remained small-scale and mostly rural endeavors until after World War II. Only a few renegade employer- or union-controlled service or group practice plans survived the interwar years (Starr 1982:305, 318–20). They were mostly nonprofit organizations closely linked to geographic areas and/or companies and, for the most part, free of government regulation. In a number of states, however, prepaid plans were discouraged; in others they were actually prohibited, blocked by court rulings favoring the AMA's position that professional, not consumer, control ought to prevail in any provision of health care. In general, these early roles and relations between the government and private prepaid health care plans are well captured by the terms of a segmented policy regime, except for the cases of restrictive state intervention on behalf of the AMA.

Three different ventures renewed government's interest in prepaid plans after the war. In 1946 a failing cooperative in Seattle sold its facilities to its physicians, who expanded them into the highly successful Group Health Cooperative of Puget Sound. In California the industrial magnate Henry Kaiser, faced with a declining workforce at the close of the war, opened enrollment in his Kaiser-Permanente Foundation to the public in 1948 and later expanded into other western states. And in New York City, Mayor Fiorello La Guardia initiated the New York Health Insurance Program in 1947, which covered medical services for city employees (Starr 1982:321–22). Meanwhile, in response to the growing popularity of the Kaiser plans, physicians in California organized their own prepayment plans, the first Independent Practice Associations (IPAs), which are discussed later. Although growth in these ventures was modest, by 1959 the AMA "ended official reprisal of prepaid group practice" (Starr 1982:327). Despite its lingering skepticism, the AMA adopted a "pluralistic" policy of free choice of medical plan for both physicians and patients, as long as HMOs were not "the exclusive or major means of providing health care delivery" (quoted in Campion 1984:340). The AMA noted in its official statement that it had found no evidence of lay interference in medical decisions in Kaiser or other prepaid plans. Also in 1959 the federal government adopted a similar position when it offered a prepaid health plan among the options in the newly created Federal Employee Health Benefits Program. However, although accepted as an alternative form of health care provision, prepaid plans continued to experience only modest growth.

By the time the Nixon administration began to express interest in the prepaid form of financing health care, the number of programs across the country was still few (prior to 1970 there were less than thirty, many of which were Kaiser affiliates), as was the number of subscribers. In the early 1970s President Nixon was searching for a proposal that would counteract congressional Democratic initiatives for national insurance with measures to control the spiraling health care costs that followed the passage of Medicare and Medicaid. He found it in an idea promoted by Dr. Paul Ellwood: the "health maintenance strategy" of private-sector prepaid plans. At the time, "the choice for health care policy lay between increasing public regulation on the one side and innovative efforts at reorganization and market-building on the other" (Brown 1983:269), a Hobson's choice to be sure for this administration. There was little evidence that what became known as HMOs could provide "the best" solution to the problems Nixon sought to solve. In fact, initial expectations for what HMOs could achieve were largely based on the "conjectural and unsubstantiated" claims of policy generalists (Brown 1983:269). But existing HMOs were developing a track record. Studies were showing that their costs were lower, primarily because of reduced hospital stays (Luft 1980). Moreover, this organizational form, situated in private-sector delivery, was ideologically and conceptually compatible with prevailing norms and values, although opposed by advocates of free choice of physician. By supporting and fostering these private-sector enterprises, the Nixon administration believed it could promote health care reform without massive government intervention. When the Health Maintenance Organization Act was passed in 1973, the government was set to embark on what Iglehart (1980) called an experiment in "venture capitalism" with the private sector.

The 1973 HMO Act provided for a system of federal grants and loans to stimulate the expansion of HMOs, old and new, as demonstration projects. The act itself did not contain the grounding for a shift from a segmented to an interventionist policy regime, because infusion of funds was to be a temporary stimulus. HMOs were expected to work toward the day when they would be self-sufficient and no longer depend on federal dollars to operate, an understanding that conformed to the prevailing norm of separate spheres for public assistance and private enterprise. The chances of HMO expansion were boosted by the requirement that all employers of twenty-five or more individuals offer their employees an opportunity to enroll in a qualified HMO if one was available in the area. (It was not mandatory, however, for employers to offer any health benefits.) The Office of Health Maintenance Organizations was set up in the Department of Health, Education, and Welfare (HEW) to oversee the new federal effort.

The initial response to the initiative from private providers was mixed at best. On the one hand, the act's definition of an HMO allowed for the inclusion of hybrid forms; as a result, it stimulated their development.[28] On the other hand, the act contained a number of restrictions that thwarted existing HMOs and raised the ire of the industry's giants.[29] What was particularly stinging was that many of the restrictions did not apply to the indemnity insurance plans with which HMOs were competing, thereby reducing the fair-market advantage of HMOs along with their flexibility to become competitive.

In all, the act was highly regulatory and sufficiently intrusive into the HMO concept to belie its ideological underpinnings favoring market-based solutions over government-directed routes. Thus, as government's approach to HMOs took shape during the 1970s, a shift in policy regimes occurred. In retrospect, and especially in light of the central role that HMOs later came to play in public policy, these early regulations may have provided a necessary foundation to establish the legitimacy of HMOs among policymakers. Those HMOs that survived the test were clearly able to contain costs while providing quality care. At the same time, success fertilized the seeds that were sown for a more cooperative relationship between the public and private sectors in the future.

A series of amendments commencing in 1976 corrected some of the prior ambiguities in the government's posture toward HMOs. An enhanced role for the Department of Health's Office of HMOs in assessing applications and certifying qualification improved mutual understanding of what was required of HMOs. Greater consistency in organizational forms and delivery systems resulted. Further facilitative amendments in 1978 supplemented the Carter administration's unprecedented support for the HMO idea.[30] The president's justifications, emphasizing private-sector know-how, may not have sounded like those of a liberal Democrat, but they were politically expedient. Brown (1983:362) presciently captures the early roots of the innovative role that government eventually adopted:

> In March 1978 . . . [HEW Secretary] Califano convened in Washington a highly publicized conference attended by 'over 1200 key health figures from the public and private sectors' to celebrate the advantages of HMOs and to discuss how the private sector could support and encourage them. Califano paid humble obeisance to the notables assembled; whatever government could do to promote HMOs, he confessed, the private sector could do better. These appeals to the public interest and to corporate pride were reinforced by direct appeals to organizational self-interest. Health maintenance organizations could help hold down employers' health care premiums, it was noted, and they might well prove to be the last chance to stave off direct intervention in and regulation of health care costs and delivery by the federal government.

The Carter administration's efforts to get the private sector to take the initiative in expanding health care provision included a strong, supportive funding role for government. It can therefore be interpreted not as an attempt to shift responsibility from the public to the private sector, but as an effort to increase the contribution of both sectors. However, at the end of the 1970s the policy was far from successful, with HMO growth much lower than expected. The many reasons for the initial "failure" of government policy toward HMOs may be less important in the long run, however, than the reasons for their abiding prominence in American health policy despite their initially weak impact.[31]

As Brown (1983) suggests, the Carter years provided an explicit rationale for HMOs that emphasized the role of the private sector in health care provision. This rationale conformed to President Reagan's philosophy, albeit without Carter's assumptions about the steady role of government. The Reagan administration renewed the HMO Act in 1981, expounding its market-based justification for further expansion of HMOs. Since Reagan's support did not include government funding, he brought to a close nearly a decade of investment amounting to $200 million. Also, in keeping with his administration's philosophy, the 1980s saw a relaxation in the definition and regulation of HMOs, as well as greater competitiveness in the HMO market, with a resulting shift from predominantly nonprofit to predominantly for-profit HMOs. The politics of the 1980s prompted a return to a segmented policy regime in which the government basically retreated from intervention by adopting a seemingly hands-off stance toward HMOs while maintaining a more passive supporting role. The rhetoric of the Reagan administration certainly reinforced the presumption that by being induced to perform a public function, the private sector was allowing government to recede to a more minimalist role. However, despite the rhetoric, and perhaps even despite the administration's intentions, government was actually strengthening both its links with HMOs and its ability to control the role that HMOs would play in health care. The features of these links and their consequences are most apparent in the direct use of HMOs by the Medicare and Medicaid programs.

Linking Sectors

The 1965 legislation that inaugurated the Medicare and Medicaid programs allowed established prepaid health plans to accept Medicare and Medicaid patients on the same payment basis as other providers, that is, fee-for-service, "customary, prevailing and reasonable" rates. Not surprisingly, the uptake was modest at best, because HMOs were unwilling to change one of their central features: capitation payment. In the 1972 Social Security Amendments the federal government yielded to HMOs' self-definition and adopted a capitation payment basis for Medicare and Medicaid patients in HMOs. The 1972 Act had also given the federal government the prerogative of calculating the initial amount of payment to HMOs in the

Medicare program and of periodically readjusting that amount to reflect excessive losses or profits within individual HMOs.[32] States in principle could make their own calculations for enrolling Medicaid patients in HMOs, but the complicated differences between states' monthly calculations of Medicaid eligibility and low reimbursement rates precluded much interest on the part of HMOs. The next set of amendments in 1976, restricting enrollment to federally certified HMOs and preventing HMOs from enrolling more than 50 percent of their membership from Medicare and Medicaid beneficiaries, was irrelevant: By 1980 only about 3 percent each of Medicare and Medicaid recipients were enrolled in HMOs.

With continuing reports of the cost-saving potential of HMOs, the federal government continued to try to arouse interest in this option. It even began to relax its own stringent requirements. In 1981 the allowable enrollment of Medicare and Medicaid recipients in HMOs was raised from 50 percent to 75 percent. At the same time, however, incentives for HMOs to enroll public-sector beneficiaries were dampened by a provision allowing patients to terminate their enrollment without cause. In 1984 this disenrollment option was modified.[33] Besides the regulatory method, the federal government adopted a new and different kind of facilitative effort to expand the use of HMOs. TEFRA 1982 authorized the Department of Health and Human Services (DHHS) to undertake large-scale demonstration projects of prospective capitation payment to selected HMOs under the Medicare program. The capitation rate was set as before at 95 percent of average Medicare per capita payments in the area.[34] However, because little effort went into providing information and education about the HMO option, these federal initiatives still did not substantially increase the number of Medicare enrollees: By 1990, only a little more than 3 percent of Medicare beneficiaries were enrolled in an HMO (and 5 percent of Medicaid recipients).

But more important by-products were generated. The demonstration projects enhanced the federal government's appreciation of the potential role of HMOs in health policy by confirming the value of the cost-containment methods employed by HMOs. By the mid-1980s, studies were showing that HMOs reduce costs by 10–40 percent of fee-for-service provision (Luft 1987). As a result, the federal government began to see its continuing efforts in the Medicare program as preparation for keeping some of the 16 percent of HMO enrollees who were between the ages of 45 and 64 in HMOs when

they reached Medicare's eligibility age. It also tacitly acknowledged that the current generation of those more than 65 years old
may be unmovable (PPRC 1990:208). An equally important by-product was the growing inclusion of HMOs among the options offered
by insurance companies and the increased uptake of the HMO option by subscribers throughout the 1980s, as Table 5.4 indicates.
HMO expansion was a long-standing, though tentative goal of the
federal government. Unlike the DRGs, which developed cautiously
and were intended only for the Medicare program, the HMO demonstration projects have gradually become more applicable.

The key to this more conscious, broader spread of government
initiatives on behalf of HMOs is the realization by government actors
of a common link between what HMOs were doing to contain costs
and what several other private-sector delivery systems were also
doing. Many private providers had adopted managed care as a fundamental feature of delivery and provision. Briefly, managed-care
programs apportion health care within a framework of limits. Thus,
in an HMO setting primary care physicians or GPs, who serve as a
patient's initial contact with the health care system, oversee the
patient's further access and continuing care needs. Alternatively,
such procedures as utilization review, though abstracted from more
holistic HMO contexts, can function as weak forms of managed care.
By the 1990s government reports were focusing primarily on the
benefits of managed care, which was emerging as a core underlying

TABLE 5.4 *HMO Growth—United States*

	NO. OF HMOS	MILLIONS OF MEMBERS	PERCENT OF EMPLOYEES (LARGE COMPANIES) IN		
			FEE FOR SERVICE	HMO (STAFF)	OTHER MANAGED CARE (IPA, PPO, POS)
1976	175				
1980	215	9.1			
1982	265	10.8			
1984	306	15.1			
1986	626	25.7			
1988	607	32.7			
1990	566	36.5	53	23	24 (1991)
1992	546	41.4	45	22	34
1994	556	50.0	42	26	32 (1993)

Sources: Adapted from GHAA (1994) and Freudenheim (1994:A1).

characteristic of a number of successful financing and delivery systems. Even some fee-for-service providers have adopted various forms of managed care. No longer confined to standard HMOs, managed care is now being promoted as the linchpin between cost containment and quality care. What the government is now promoting through the managed-care concept is less an organizational form than a form of behavior that applies to both organizations and individuals in them. That behavior is self-management or self-regulation, applied in accordance with social standards of efficient and effective health care. The transition to greater acceptance of managed care by the government in the United States includes a subtle change still in its infancy, one that no longer focuses simply on the value of managed care in cost reduction but also recognizes its effectiveness in health care. This newfound appreciation is informed no doubt by findings that managed care may not actually reduce costs as much as redistribute expenditures toward more efficient and effective care (Wallack 1991). As articulated in a government report: "physicians, patients, insurers, and managed-care organizations share accountability for improving outcomes of patient care and for meeting cost-containment objectives" (PPRC 1992:313–14).

Whether or not the promise is illusory depends on the role of the federal government, acting as central coordinator and overseer of utilization practices and quality assurance. Without these, managed care becomes nothing more than price discounting, and accordingly, it raises concerns about incentives to underserve. The DHHS and the Health Care Financing Administration (HCFA) are currently developing demonstration projects on utilization, quality, and related features of managed care for the Medicare and Medicaid programs.[35] OBRA 1990 authorized these projects in the hope of encouraging beneficiaries of the public programs to use managed-care plans and in the hope of promoting their use among all providers. Most important among HCFA's recommendations are the development of community health centers and managed-care programs for Medicaid recipients,[36] and the development of a Health Care Quality Improvement System—a quality assurance guidance program that is intentionally similar to systems used in the private sector (PPRC 1993:260). Without the standardization provided by the Health Care Quality Improvement System, managed care for Medicaid recipients runs the risk of being second-class care. If the system is utilized across private-sector programs, it will reinforce the role of managed care in unifying the provision of health care in the United States.

Early results from the demonstrations were encouraging. Compared to fee-for-service Medicaid recipients, those in the managed-care demonstration projects were as satisfied and received comparable care at lower costs for the states (PPRC 1992, chapter 6). Some underserving did occur, however, in the managed-care settings, and visible deficiencies for Medicaid recipients occurred in both types of payment systems (for example, for prenatal care). To develop safeguards against underserving and to foster joint understanding of standards, protocols for treatment, quality controls, and referral guarantees, HCFA is strengthening annual review procedures, requiring that these be conducted both internally and by independent external committees. The Health Care Quality Improvement System is the major implementation tool. What is unique about current efforts is the strong federal oversight role and active state monitoring. Such coordination between these two units of government was formerly absent in the Medicaid program. At the same time, HCFA is entering new areas of collaboration with the private sector. It is working with independent external review organizations on standardizing principles to guide evaluations of managed-care programs. Demonstration projects in the Health Care Quality Improvement System program and evaluations of them are being funded jointly by HCFA and the Kaiser Family Foundation. To allow states to implement portions of the program as they acquire the capability, the Health Care Quality Improvement System program is not mandatory at present. But HCFA foresees the eventual development of national standards and enforcement as well as a shift in focus away from process toward outcome measures once national standards are implemented.

President Clinton's health care plan put managed care at the center of a solution to reform health care delivery and cost control. The failure of his plan does not signify a retreat from managed care. In fact, the private sector is continuing to incorporate managed-care programs among its options and to encourage greater use of managed care. By 1993, 75 percent of all physicians had an arrangement with a managed-care plan. It is interesting that the growth of managed care occurred in part because of the "threat" of federal government intervention (as suggested in President Clinton's proposals), which was enough to spur the private sector into action. Experimentation with managed care has so far confirmed its future role in American health care. The uptake of the HMO option also seems to have contributed to a slowdown in the rate of growth in national health care expenditures (Levit et al. 1994).

Activities on the part of the federal government in promoting and supporting HMO growth in the private sector are not well captured by the terms of either a segmented or an interventionist policy regime framework. The federal government has not transferred responsibility to local or private-sector actors. Yet its involvement, although regulatory, is not intrusive. The federal government is attempting to coordinate the activities of a number of different actors and to facilitate the construction among them of a common purpose—that health care costs be controlled without jeopardizing the quantity and quality of care. At present, government actors have been advancing the cost control part more forcefully. Were their efforts embedded in a prototypical integrative policy regime, the construction of social goals would be less intensely guided by single-minded objectives. As government actors yield to the reality of potential (but inevitable) contradictions between the tenets of cost control and high-quality health care, they may join other actors on a more equal footing, collaborating to sort out and redirect future developments in American health care.

Conclusion

My task in this chapter has been to understand the consequences of privatization as it is unfolding in the health care systems of the three countries. I have noted that the state has not handed over responsibility to the private sector, nor are state actors using their regulatory powers to enforce private-sector compliance with public standards. What is most noteworthy about the decision making currently under way is the mutual give and take between public and private goals and preferred means. The result is a negotiated order of health care. Therefore, we are witnessing neither a return to segmented roles and relations nor relentless state interventions; instead we are seeing the possible emergence of an integrative policy regime.

There is no doubt that privatization endangers equity in any area of social provision. Each country has had to define the limits of acceptable inequalities that inevitably result from increased market forces in health care and has had to determine the extent to which government regulation can enforce these limits. In all three countries the state has called on the private sector to accept an obligation for health care and to contribute services while restraining private interests. The state has also provided an arena for the construction of a common understanding of basic health care and modalities for achieving greater equality. In the process, it has ceded some of its own powers for the sake of broader provision. Most important, it has insisted that the health care outcome represent an improvement in the status quo ante. These consequences do not suggest a reduction in the role of the state. In fact, if true, they support the possibility of an increase in the capacity of the state to oversee a broader base of social provision.

NOTES

1. For an earlier treatise on problems in public-sector accountability, see Smith and Hague, eds. (1971).

2. Estimates indicate that half of Britain's private paying patients are not residents (Calnan, Cant, Gabe 1993:2).

3. Abortions are legal in Britain but must compete for scarce resources within the NHS. Therefore, approximately half of all UK residents receiving abortions pay for themselves in the private sector (Laing and Buisson 1988–1989:36).

4. For 1988 the value of private-sector care was estimated at £1 billion and the value of private insurance sales was estimated at £750 million, with claims paid amounting to £615 million (Propper 1989:2–3). In the same period the NHS revenue budget was £11,539 million and its capital budget was £766 million. This means that the value of private-sector health care is approximately one-twelfth the value of the NHS. A different source estimates the 1987 total value of the for-profit private and nonprofit voluntary sectors as £4,410 million (Laing and Buisson 1988–1989:1), and £7306 million in 1990 (Laing and Buisson 1992:62).

5. The rate of growth in private-sector health care rose from 10 percent or under prior to 1979 to 30 percent in 1980 and 38 percent in 1982. Thereafter, however, the rate of growth declined to 16 percent in 1983 and 8 percent in 1987.

6. Major public assets in utilities and transportation were also sold, or otherwise denationalized. (See also Heald [1988].)

7. The number of policyholders rose from 1.1 million in 1978 to 2 million in 1984 (Laing and Buisson 1988–1989:42). The actual number of people covered is estimated to be approximately twice as large, because many policies are for families.

8. Approximately four times as many individuals in professional groups have private insurance as in the population as a whole (Laing and Buisson 1988–1989:46). Three percent of skilled manual and 2 percent of unskilled manual workers have private health insurance, compared with 34 percent of people aged 45–64 in professional occupations (Calnan, Cant, Gabe 1993:3).

9. In 1989, 54 percent of the privately insured were in company schemes, 24 percent were in individual plans, and 18 percent were in group schemes.

10. Of these only 25 percent of the premiums are wholly paid by employers and another 14 percent are partly paid (Laing and Buisson 1988–1989:50). An interesting development within the private insurance system in Britain is the movement away from direct reimbursement of providers (that is, from an essentially retrospective system with no controls on price) to direct negotiations between insurers and providers to determine prospective rates of reimbursement. In addition, insurers have begun to persuade providers to limit their price in exchange for inclusion on a "preferred list" of specialists and hospitals, not too unlike the American Preferred Provider Organizations (PPOs) (OECD 1992:118).

11. Private hospitals were placed under local authority planning controls. Only proposals for surgical facilities, for facilities with more than 120 beds, and for expansions that would add more than 20 percent over three years to the number of beds in a district are subject to approval by the secretary of state for health.

12. In 1990 the charge was £3.05 per prescription or £43.50 for a "season's ticket" purchased annually and prospectively.

13. In 1980 the DHSS specified certain ethical and behavioral principles to safeguard the interests of NHS patients in those facilities and with those physicians catering to pay-bed patients. The nonstatutory principles are outlined in Chandra and Kakabadse (1985:12).

14. The private sector regards NHS beds as "unfair competition" because they are cheaper than private-pay beds (Mohan and Woods 1985:209).

15. DHSS, letter from the minister of health (Dr. Gerard Vaughn), August 20, 1981, reproduced in Chandra and Kakabadse (1985:85). The circular on which this letter was based identified three potential areas where contractual arrangements might be used: (1) short-term contracts to overcome temporary difficulties in the provision of NHS services (for example, to tackle long waiting lists or to maintain a certain level of services while NHS facilities are closed for building work); (2) medium-term contracts (for example, before new capital facilities become available); (3) long-term contracts enabling more effective use of total resources (Chandra and Kakabadse 1985:53).

16. Weller and Manga (1983:496) claim that in the early 1980s the medical profession in Canada was "clearly in the vanguard of the fight for the reprivatization of health."

17. Private hospital insurance began in Canada in the 1930s and spread rapidly in the 1940s and 1950s. Private insurance for medical care appeared later and spread more slowly. Just prior to the introduction of the first stage of the national program, one-half of the population had private coverage for both medical and surgical care. (See Evans [1984].)

18. Seventy-five percent of total institutional long-term care facilities are

for-profit and they contain more than 50 percent of the beds, indicating that they are smaller and less "institutional" than the public and charitable facilities (Forbes, Jackson, Krause 1987, chapter 2).

19. The province extends both deficit funding and per diem funding for public and charitable facilities, but only per diem funding for proprietary facilities (Tarman 1990:45). Once provincial regulation and funding were in place, the provincial government assumed the right to inspect facilities. Scandals in the 1970s and 1980s brought to public attention the fact that private facilities, where recipients "pay for what they get," are more capable of skimping on care in order to maintain profit and getting away with it.

20. In 1993 the figure was set at $35 (Cdn) per day, an amount that everyone can afford insofar as everyone receives a pension.

21. Once a physician certifies that an elderly person requires, for example, meals on wheels in order to remain at home, that service is provided free of charge in principle, depending on availability in the community. The provincial government reimburses the provider directly. (See Ministry of Community and Social Services, Ministry of Health, and Ministry of Citizenship [1991].)

22. The idea of incentives and the freedom to determine the specific forms of savings as well as their use are similar to what occurs in Britain's hospital trusts and among fundholding GPs and local health authorities. It also resembles the thinking behind the American DRGs.

23. Between 1976 and 1986 the bed occupancy rate in public general hospitals rose from 77 percent to 83 percent (MacLean and Mix 1991).

24. Hospital productivity is measured by "cost per patient day." The very large increases in hospital costs are bound to create declines in the measure of productivity. Using aggregate data for public general hospitals, MacLean and Mix (1991) found that between 1976 and 1986 hospital productivity declined by 19.8 percent. When inpatient and outpatient services were separated, inpatient service productivity declined by 16.3 percent; outpatient service productivity declined by 2.3 percent.

25. Similar questions were raised in all three countries. (See Evans [1983] and Culyer and Meads [1992].)

26. The Medicare and Medicaid programs can be said to coopt the private sector for public purposes in that private actors must conform to the terms of the public program, which is especially problematical with regard to reimbursement levels. However, private providers have not been coopted into serving these programs to the extent that they find ways of "gaming the system" or opting out. It can also be argued that the base for the government's calculation of its reimbursement levels is determined by providers' fees or willingness to comply. If the consequence of low levels of reimbursement is less care for the recipients of Medicare and Medicaid, providers can still be said to set the rules of the game. Therefore, a kind of double cooptation pertains: The government engages private providers on terms set by the providers but restricts providers' freedom vis-à-vis public-sector recipients of health care.

27. Another appropriate case study would be insurance reform. (For a summary of the government's activities and private-sector responses, see PPRC [1994, 1995].) On the assumption of universal, mandated coverage based on private-sector insurance competition, the commission recommended that certain

basic rules be adopted: a standard benefit package, coordinated open seasons for enrollment, limits on marketing techniques, a guarantee that plans accept everyone regardless of health status, community rating, and risk-adjusted payments to plans (PPRC 1994:109). However, without knowing more about the role of the state in overseeing these rules, we cannot say what kind of policy framework would structure their implementation. The commission also recommended that "a national entity be created to make the most important coverage decisions" and to maintain a list of services and indications that are included in a "national standard benefits package" (PPRC 1994:229).

28. The traditional prepaid plans that had been developing for decades combined financing and delivery in one organization with a limited number (and therefore choice) of physicians working fully for the plan, usually on a salary basis. The HMO Act applied the notion of prepaid to subscribers but not providers and thereby included Independent Practice Associations (IPAs) as types of HMOs. IPAs are third-party payer plans with discounted fee-based services provided in private offices on a contract basis. There is little difference at present between IPAs and another hybrid, Preferred Provider Organizations (PPOs), except in their contractual affiliations. Some prepaid plans allow patients to choose "out-of-network" physicians at a higher price and on an indemnity insurance basis. These are usually "point of service" decisions, from which their name (POS) is derived.

29. Traditional HMOs offer comprehensive services, but the mix varied across HMOs. The legislation specified a package of basic benefits that included dental care for children, mental health, home health, and alcoholism services but excluded vision care, physical therapy, and prescription drugs, which either disqualified some existing HMOs or encouraged them to reduce their comprehensive coverage. In addition, HMOs were required to base their premiums on community rating and to permit open enrollment, which some, but not all, were already doing.

30. Among others, there were changes in the mandated benefit package, relaxation of the open-enrollment requirement, higher ceilings for grant awards, extension of the loan eligibility period, establishment of an HMO management training program and a technical assistance authority (Iglehart 1980:665). The community-rating requirement was not modified until 1988, when HMOs were allowed to adjust rates prospectively to take into account the medical conditions of specific groups, with some restrictions (Langwell 1990:74).

31. See Brown (1983) for a full analysis of the reasons for failure, both of government policy and of HMOs during this period.

32. The initial calculation was based on a percentage (95 percent) of average Medicare fee-for-service payments in the geographical area (called an adjusted average per capita cost). Further adjustments allowed each HMO to retain 5 percent of its savings (any additional profits were to be returned to Medicare) but required the HMO to absorb its losses fully. These early contracts were called "risk" based, reflecting the uncertainty of the venture for both the government and HMOs. Although this nomenclature is still employed, I use the generic term *capitation payment.*

33. During the first month patients can disenroll at any time, thereafter they must remain in the HMO for at least five months. Medicaid recipients, however, remain subject to loss of eligibility on a monthly basis. One study found that at the end of a thirty-two-month period, only 44 percent of Medicaid recipients remained eligible for the entire period (discussed in PPRC 1992:169).

34. This payment was sometimes more than the amount charged by the HMO, in which case the HMO was required to reduce patient copayment charges or increase the benefits offered to Medicare patients. Where the payment was lower than the HMO's normal fee, the uptake was minimal (PPRC 1990:209).

35. For these demonstration projects HCFA is authorized to waive basic requirements of state Medicaid programs for freedom of choice, uniform statewide operation, and comparability of benefits. There are three principal types of waivers: program waivers under Section 1915 of the Social Security Act, congressionally mandated demonstrations, and demonstration waivers granted under Section 1115 of the Social Security Act (PPRC 1995:156). (Also see Holahan et al. [1995].)

36. Although only some states have taken the initiative to encourage or even mandate HMO use by Medicaid recipients, the increase has been greater than that among Medicare recipients. In 1991, 5.01 percent of HMO enrollees were Medicaid recipients, and in 1993, 8.67 percent. In contrast, in 1991, 5.82 percent of HMO enrollees were Medicare recipients, and were in 1993, 7.16 percent (HCIA 1994:xxi). The PPRC realizes that improved access for Medicaid recipients also requires greater equity in physicians' fees for Medicaid and Medicare patients, whether according to a fee schedule or capitation payment system. The initial Medicaid capitation rate has been set at 90 to 100 percent of average Medicaid fee-for-service rates in an area, even though Medicaid rates are 64 percent of Medicare rates (PPRC 1992:169).

Chapter Six

Health Care in the Welfare State

At an empirical level of analysis the differences in the health care systems of Britain, Canada, and the United States take on very real significance for providers and recipients alike. Britain's national health service is centralized; it is currently undergoing major administrative decentralization that is expected to ease some bottlenecks in provision. Canada has a national insurance system with provincial implementation, in which patients are waiting longer for certain surgeries and returning to their physicians more frequently for shorter visits. The United States has a mix of public insurance programs, public service programs, and a predominant private insurance system, all of which leaves 16 percent of the population uninsured. This chapter summarizes several of the empirical differences among the three health care systems. But it also analyzes their elements of commonality.

In previous chapters I have shown that fundamental similarities among the three health care systems exist at relatively high levels of abstraction. First, I have indicated that Britain, Canada, and the United States are all liberal welfare states. In contrast to the sort of state intervention that we see in social democratic systems, liberal welfare states lean toward market solutions to social problems and place greater emphasis on individuals' rights and freedoms than on the needs of the collectivity. Developments in any one component of a welfare state, such as health policy, may deviate somewhat from prototypical characteristics or the overall trends in a country's social policy nexus.[1] Nevertheless, recent changes in privatization in the three countries under study suggest that reliance on market solutions remains significant.[2]

Second, I have outlined in previous chapters a similar evolution in the policy regimes organizing the three health care systems. That Britain, Canada, and the United States are liberal welfare states accounts for the fundamental hold of a segmented policy regime in all of them. This regime type entails a separation between the domains of state versus market or public versus private sectors. I also argued in previous chapters that state intervention becomes deeper than intended in liberal welfare states. Governments in Britain, Canada, and the United States have constructed weighty networks of regulatory measures that constitute interventionist policy regimes. These similarities hold despite the empirical differences in the three health care systems.

Analyses of similarities despite differences and vice versa commonly focus on the familiar state-versus-market dimension. Many studies of social policies in Britain, Canada, and the United States conclude that of the three countries, Britain is the most state-oriented and the United States is the most market-oriented. This conclusion is neither enlightening nor altogether valid. In fact, the state-versus-market axis and the additional polarities it entails (such as regulation versus competition) are too simplistic to capture the complexities of public- and private-sector roles in health care. Previous chapters have shown that a new relationship is evolving among health care actors that in some ways transcends such dualistic characterization. The policy regimes framework offers an alternative conceptualization of the policy process, one that focuses less on market and state than on principles and norms of roles, relations, and decision making. Market and state factors are included in the basic principles and norms of policy regimes, but only along with other factors, such as respect for tradition or for professional authority. Its inclusiveness grants the policy regimes framework greater potential for tapping the complexity of evolving social relations.

A full appreciation of emerging forms cannot be based solely on the single axis between state and market that has informed so much of our theorizing about the welfare state. We must conceptualize more fully the gray area in mid-axis and posit a third dimension to clarify the nature of the multiple tensions involved in the process of social change. The literature on the welfare state offers several formulations of a third dimension for analyzing social policies.

Titmuss (1963) first developed two models of welfare, which he called residual and institutional redistributive, that correspond to the market-versus-state dimensions of social organization. He then constructed an industrial achievement-performance model based on the work ethic as a third alternative (1974). In his third model, social welfare institutions act as adjuncts of the economy, and needs are met on the basis of merit, work performance, and productivity. Titmuss's formulations are applicable to, for example, pension schemes, which in many welfare states operate on the basis of contributory social insurance. Overall, Titmuss's model of an industrial achievement-performance welfare system is conceptually very close to the normative premises of the residual model. It is therefore less well developed than his other two types.

Following along similar lines of analysis, Esping-Andersen (1990) adds a number of considerations to Titmuss's conceptual framework. He distinguishes three clusters of regime types, two of which—the liberal and social democratic welfare states—are standard fare and roughly approximate the market-versus-state dimension of analysis. His third regime cluster, a corporatist welfare state, approximates the social democratic in extent and depth of social provision. There is one difference: Corporatist welfare states, Esping-Andersen (1985) claims, maintain class and status distinctions, so that their redistributive effects are negligible. His formulation of this type derives from his earlier thoughts on paternalistic or conservative welfare states that tend toward compulsory insurance plans based on contributions, the archetype being Germany. (For a similar triad, see Bunce and Hicks [1987].)

Hage and Hanneman (1980) develop three "paradigms" of welfare state growth. The first two conform to established theories: the functionalist paradigm, driven by "changes in needs of populations and resource constraints" (p. 46), and the pluralist paradigm, constituted by political interest group mobilization and

competition. They call their third approach the cybernetic paradigm, in which the "degree of responsiveness of the state is dependent upon its awareness of social welfare needs and is limited by
its internal structure" (p. 48). In this model the state engages in
extensive knowledge-seeking activities. Variations in the organizational abilities of states to transform knowledge into implementation of social welfare programs distinguish strong states
from weak states.

These typologies, together with those presented in chapter 1,
share a similar orientation—all strive to express something other
than state-based and market-based forms of organization, without
completely discarding the prototypes. The authors commonly
select those features of state- and market-based typologies that are
pertinent to the particular issue they study. Then, with additional
considerations and modifications, they form a new whole. This
endeavor spans the social sciences in general (cf. Lindblom 1977;
Alford and Friedland 1985; Powell 1990).

I too have developed a new concept, integrative policy regime, to
capture a third dimension of analysis that seeks to modify and
recast certain features of the state-versus-market dichotomy. A
main difference between an integrative policy regime and the third-
type alternative just discussed is my emphasis on process rather
than on institutional outcome. Among my tasks has been deci-
phering how integration comes about: What are its agencies and its
patterns of evolution? Who chooses the features that are extracted
from segmented and interventionist policy regimes? And how are
those features altered so that they constitute a new integrative policy regime? I do not in the end fall back on known power holders as
the main conduits of change. In fact, I emphasized in the chapters
on individual countries that in its new role the state does not
impose a predetermined agenda, nor in their new roles do physicians dominate decision making. I have focused on collaboration as
the core process of constructing a negotiated social order based on
mutual give and take. The third dimension of welfare state change
that is a central concern of this study emerges from an examination
of what drives and restrains the actions of providers and recipients
of health care, especially when the causes of social action are not
clearly embedded in state or market dimensions alone, and when
social actors resort to neither the rationalities nor the contending
interests central to the state-versus-market dichotomies of social

action. My concept of integrative policy regime is suggestive. I claim not that it currently exists but that it may be emerging. What is currently discernible, I have noted throughout, is a coexistence among policy regimes. Persisting features of segmented or interventionist policy regimes create tensions that lend themselves to resolutions based on collaborative processes.

State and Market

Let us first consider the three health care systems in terms of the state versus market axis. We will see immediately that what appears to be true on the surface is not so upon closer analysis. Take the familiar theme that because both Britain and Canada have national health care, their systems are more state determined and the American system is more market determined. Important qualifications appear when the concepts of state and market are scrutinized empirically.

The State

Decomposing the state along a centralized–decentralized axis yields a perspective of the state as a more complex actor. In all three countries there is significant decentralization in the role of the state, challenging the assumption that the United States is more decentralized or less state oriented than Britain or Canada. Ironically, the regulatory framework shows the state in the United States to be more microinterventionist than in the other two countries, which, once their macroframeworks are established, assume a less persistently visible presence.

The British National Health Service (NHS) is organized hierarchically with a functional division of labor among the levels of government that grants considerable program determination to the district health authorities (DHAs). Changes currently under way in Britain allow greater purchasing power to DHAs as well as to self-governing hospital trusts and independent, fundholding general practitioners (GPs), thereby introducing marketlike factors, such as competition, into government activities. Decisions about the particulars of spending are now highly decentralized in Britain, granting the DHAs considerable discretion over what level and kind of services they purchase. At the same time, however, overall funding for health care continues to be highly centralized in the Treasury. The centralized–decentralized state axis is thus constituted by a division of decision-making labor, such that the central level is responsible for macrobudgetary decisions, and the decentralized level for the specifics of health care. The substantive decisions of the state are pushed far down the line in Britain.

In Canada the provinces administer the health insurance system and construct their own legislation within the national framework of the Canada Health Act, which sets basic guidelines for delivery and provision. Variations among the provinces are minor (especially when compared to the significant differences among the states in the U.S. Medicaid program). The federal government's contribution to provincial health care budgets is indexed to national economic growth. But the fiscal power of the federal government is constrained because its portion of total expenditures is lower than provincial government expenditures. The Canada Health Act of 1984 is the only national legislation in that country. The provincial governments legislate many regulations, but these are not as microinterventionist as comparable government directives in the United States. (Recall the differences between the terms of the Medicare Fee Schedule in the United States and the provincial government/professional association negotiations over fee-for-service reimbursement in Canada.) To be sure, there is also a huge difference in the reach of government and the proportion of medical services affected in these countries. But the analytical point here pertains to the role of government, not to its quantitative output. In part, the global budgeting systems in both Britain and Canada reduce governments' requirements for detailed reports, and the unit-based funding in the United States (the most common unit is medical procedure, as in the Medicare Fee Schedule) increases the demand for stricter accounting of expenditures. In part too, nationalized systems reduce administration in general and its accompanying thirst for information.

In the United States the Veteran's Administration and the Medicare program (for the elderly) are centrally regulated, and their (circumscribed) universal eligibility criteria make them directly comparable to the national programs of Britain and Canada. The federal government issues minimum standard regulations for Medicaid (for the poor). These regulations have become increasingly more specific over the years, but there remains considerable variation in Medicaid coverage and service provision across the fifty states. As elaborated in the preceding chapters on individual countries, the United States is more burdened with multiple microinterventionist measures at both federal and state levels of government than the other two countries (recall, for example, CONs and DRGs). The burden of administration in the United States is particularly heavy when we include the role of the private sector, especially the myriad insurance companies (GAO 1991:28–29, 40; Evans et al. 1989).

Besides these differences in regulation, the state's fiscal role differs in the three countries, with important consequences for depictions of state-versus-market orientations. Both the British and Canadian systems are financed largely out of general taxation;[3] in the United States only the Veterans' Administration, Medicaid, and parts of Medicare are funded out of general taxation. Table 6.1 compares the overall distribution of taxation in the three countries. It indicates that although the United States derives less of its revenue from taxation, the cumulative toll of taxes in Britain and Canada is not as great as American folklore would have us believe. Note, for instance, that the contribution of personal income tax to total tax receipts is lowest in Britain and that disposable family income is a higher percentage of gross pay in both Britain and Canada than in the United States, due in part to the contribution of family assistance programs. The higher rate of taxation on goods and services (including medical goods and services) in Britain is a problem, especially because the lowest personal tax rate is relatively high. Also note that social security contributions in the United States are much higher than in the other two countries, partly because of the Medicare program, which is funded through a combination of employer and employee contributions to the Social Security Fund, government contributions, and individual beneficiary contributions (premiums, deductibles, copayments). The fiscal role of the state is highly visible in the United States and appears to be no less overbearing than in Britain or Canada.

Perhaps the most perplexing financing dilemma in the United States is its high expenditures for health care. Table 6.2 indicates that as a percentage of GDP both Britain and Canada spend less on health care than the United States spends.[4] These expenditures must be understood within the broader framework of develop-

TABLE 6.1 *Taxation**

	TOTAL TAX RECEIPTS % OF GDP	TAX STRUCTURES AS % OF TOTAL TAX RECEIPTS						RATE STRUCTURES OF CENTRAL GOVERNMENT PERSONAL INCOME TAX		DISPOSABLE INCOME OF AVERAGE PRODUCTION WORKER AS % OF GROSS PAY	
		PERSONAL INCOME TAX	CORPORATE INCOME TAX	SOCIAL SECURITY CONTRIBUTIONS		GOODS AND SERVICES	OTHER TAXES	LOWEST RATE %	HIGHEST RATE %	SINGLE PERSON	MARRIED WITH TWO CHILDREN[†]
				EMPLOYEES	EMPLOYERS						
Britain	36.7	28.4	11.0	6.6	10.0	30.4	13.6	25.0	40.0	73.5	83.1
Canada	37.1	40.8	6.8	4.3	9.7	27.4	11.0	17.0	29.0	75.5	86.8
United States	29.9	35.8	7.3	11.6	16.6	16.5	12.2	15.0	28.0	73.6	80.9

*1990.

[†]Takes account of family allowances and/or tax reliefs.

Source: Adapted from OECD (1993:42–43).

TABLE 6.2 *Health Care Expenditures, Total*

	% GDP				PER CAPITA*	PERCENT PUBLIC			PERCENT PRIVATE		
	1975	1980	1990	1992	1992	1975	1980	1990	1975	1980	1990
Britain	5.5	5.8	6.0	7.1	$1,151	91.1	89.6	83.5	8.9	10.4	16.5
Canada	7.3	7.4	9.3	10.3	1,949	76.4	74.7	72.6	23.6	25.3	27.4
United States	8.4	8.4	12.5	13.6	3,094	41.5	42.0	42.4	58.5	58.0	57.6

*U.S. dollars.

Source: Adapted from OECD (1992b:22) and Schieber, Poullier, and Greenwald (1994:101–102).

ments in other social programs, especially unemployment, old age assistance, and family assistance.[5] Low expenditures in any one policy area are often related to high expenditures in another, especially if low expenditures do not fully meet needs that are then absorbed in another area. Alternatively, high expenditures in one area may permit low expenditures in another. For example, it can be argued that the United States spends more on welfare than other countries because it does not spend enough on labor market training and housing.

Within the larger picture of public-sector expenditure, we note in table 6.3 that Canada devotes more public funding than Britain or the United States to all social programs except pensions, which are proportionately highest in the United States. Figure 6.1 demonstrates that the sum of social expenditure is lowest in the United States. Thus, among the many reasons for the higher health care expenditures in the United States may be the nation's inability to reduce the gap between rich and poor (despite higher expenditures on education).[6] This is another way of saying that if the purpose of social expenditure is to alleviate poverty, social expenditure in the United States has been inefficient. It is also possible that because Britain and Canada spend more on social programs overall, they both spend less on health care per se.

The Market

What about the complementary role of the market, which is currently changing in all three countries? When compared to the size of the public sector, the private-sector contribution to health care is growing in both Britain and Canada and is shrinking slightly in the United States (see table 6.2). The composition of relative sector roles in health care varies considerably among the three countries, however. In Britain the private sector includes supplementary

TABLE 6.3 *Social Expenditures (public sector)*

| | SOCIAL PROGRAMS (% GDP), 1985 | | | |
	EDUCATION	HEALTH	PENSIONS	UNEMPLOYMENT
Britain	5.0	5.2	6.7	1.8
Canada	5.9	6.4	5.4	3.3
United States	5.3	4.4	7.2	0.4

Source: Adapted from OECD (1988:11).

insurance purchased by both individuals and employers (approximately 10 percent of the population currently carries some form of private insurance), and private hospital corporations (8 percent of acute hospital beds are private) (OECD 1992a:116). Britain has introduced increasingly greater charges for prescription drugs, medical devices, and dental care, but the amounts are still nominal compared to the noninsured costs for these items in the other two countries.

In Canada the private sector includes out-of-pocket payments for services and benefits not covered by the public program, and/or payments for supplementary health insurance for these items (private hospital beds, prescriptions drugs, medical devices, dental care). Both employers and individuals purchase supplementary insurance in Canada on a more widespread basis than in Britain. Canadians also purchase private nursing home care, some of which is for profit. Hospitals in Canada are in principle publicly owned, but they are sometimes considered to be private and nonprofit because they are governed by lay boards of trustees. Most hospital funding in Canada comes from (provincial) government sources. Some private capital fundraising for hospitals also occurs, especially for the purchase of advanced diagnostic tech-

FIGURE 6.1   *Social Expenditures, Public Sector (as % of GDP)*

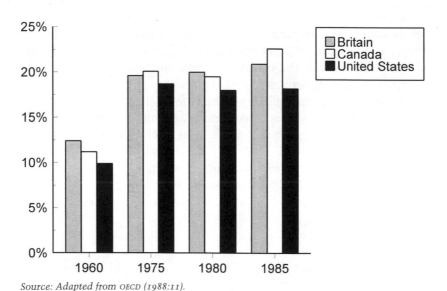

Source: Adapted from OECD (1988:11).

nology. User fees for services and benefits covered by the public program, as well as extra billing by physicians (charges to patients over and above government reimbursement rates), have been banned in Canada.

The components of the private sector in the United States are too vast to name; it is more concise to say that in the main the public sector consists of the administration and financing of part of the Medicare and Medicaid programs. Insofar as the public contribution to Medicaid in particular is much lower than providers' costs, private subsidization occurs. Similarly, insofar as the uninsured in the United States are treated in hospital emergency rooms, taxpayers' dollars, for one, subsidize such care. The public sector also includes the Veterans Administration, insurance policies of public employees, and municipal or county hospitals. Since a lower proportion of the population is covered by insurance (public and private) in the United States than in the other two countries, out-of-pocket expenses are greater. The available data indicate that individual payments for health care are greatest in the United States, followed at some distance by Canada. Another indicator of the greater reliance on private purchasing in the United States is the relative proportion of Medicare recipients (over 30 percent) purchasing Medigap insurance compared with the number of elderly buying private insurance in Britain and Canada. Although all the elderly in the United States are covered by Medicare, its coverage is limited. Chapter 5 elaborated the theme that close examination of privatization shows it to be a complex phenomenon in all three countries, and not easily captured by simple contrasts.

Regulation or Competition?

The information presented thus far might be, and has been, used to say that, regardless of nuances in regulations, taxation, and expenditures, Britain has managed to exercise greater control over rising health care costs because the role of the state overpowers market factors, unlike the situation in the United States. The argument is reinforced when we note that recent increases in health care expenditures in Britain coincide with a loosening of central control in favor of competition at the local level. Furthermore, because in Britain the state performs both funding and management functions to a far greater extent than in Canada or the United States, its centralized regulatory power is greater than in the other two countries. I have suggested, in contrast, that centralization and regulation were more critical tools in the exercise of state authority in the past than in the present. The case of Britain illustrates well how competitive marketlike forces as well as decentralization have entered health care and transformed social relations. However, in none of the three countries are we witnessing a swing along the axis from state to market, because in all of them the introduction of marketlike factors is occurring within a continuing strong framework of government regulation. In preceding chapters, I indicated that the increasing role of the private sector or of marketlike factors in health care could suggest a retreat to a segmented policy regime. Government leaders use the vocabulary of separate domains to justify policy changes, claiming that the state had overreached its boundaries and that the private sector should pick up where the state left off. At the same time, however, unintended consequences are appearing as the state continues to regulate many of the activities in health care provision. The conceptual trap involved in the question "What is occurring, regulation or competition?" cannot be broken in terms of the state-versus-market axis. As social actors in Britain, Canada, and the United States engage in cost control efforts, they are turning to alternative methods and reference points, which I have attempted to capture within the concept of an integrative policy regime. I now elaborate some of these alternatives.

The Role of Providers

Despite the variations in overall expenditures discussed thus far, all the countries under consideration have decided that health care costs and expenditures are rising too much and too fast, and that forms of control other than those used in the past are necessary. All three countries have engaged in a number of strategies to control different dimensions of health care expenditures, and all have identified clinical autonomy and overuse of hospitals and technology as two main areas ripe for control. Table 6.4 summarizes the strategies of cost containment being undertaken in each country. In many cases they rest less on state intervention than on negotiations between state and social actors.

TABLE 6.4 *Cost Control Strategies*

	DEMAND	RESOURCES		PHYSICIANS	PHYSICIAN PAYMENT	COMPETITION
		HOSPITALS	TECHNOLOGY			
Britain	GP as gatekeeper; Some small user fees	Global budgeting, national to district levels; Community clinics; Other community care	At hospital level, separate budget; Rationing at discretion of physician	National government control of supply (education, distribution); Medical audits by profession	Capitation (GPs); Salary (consultants)	Contracting out for some services; Decentralized budget-holding for some hospitals and GPs; Private supplementary insurance; Part-time NHS consultant contracts
Canada	Limits on number of services, by province; No coverage for private rooms, dental care, medical aids, etc.	Global budgeting, provincial level; Community clinics, mostly in Quebec	Separate capital budgets, acquisition approval required	Provincial government control of medical school places; Provincial utilization reviews by lay boards; Practice guidelines by profession	Fee-for-service; Total increase negotiated at provincial level; Fee schedules developed by provincial medical associations	Among private supplementary insurances; Some private nursing homes; Some contract management of hospitals
U. S.	Public: Medicare: premiums, etc.; specified limits on hospital days, etc. Medicaid: physician discretion. Private: Private insurance: premiums, etc.; specified limits. HMOs: GP as gatekeeper; limited physician choice	DRGs (prospective); Public and Private: CONs; State planning agencies	Public and Private: CONs; State planning agencies	PROs; Practice guidelines; Practice guidelines	Medicare: Fee-for-service; Medicare Fee Schedule; Medicaid: Fee-for-service variable % of rate; Private insurance: Fee-for-service (retrospective); HMOs: Mixed: mostly salary, some discounted fee-for-service	Some contracting out for services

Physicians

Differences in the supply and distribution of physicians account for many of the disparities in the delivery of health care services in the three countries. As figure 6.2 shows, the United States has the greatest overall ratio of physicians to population. Medical organizations in the United States have at times predicted impending physician shortages, a worry not confirmed by the aggregate data. The relatively high figure for physician supply in Canada has caused concern about overservicing in that country. Britain's relative undersupply of physicians is striking but not alarming, considering the greater reliance on nonphysician medical and paramedical personnel.

As important for service provision as overall numbers is the ratio of general practitioners (GPs) and specialists. Canada maintains the highest ratio of GPs to specialists (53 to 47), and some Canadian provinces (for example, Ontario) have a guideline policy aiming at a ratio of 55 to 45. Considering that all British residents must register with a GP and cannot see a specialist without a referral, it is surprising that there are fewer GPs than specialists in Britain (40 to 60). The data on which figure 6.2 is based include within the category "physicians" all hospital staff consultants, over half of whom are junior hospital doctors. If one discounts both GP trainees and consultant trainees, the ratio is reversed: 64 GPs to

FIGURE 6.2   *Physician Supply*

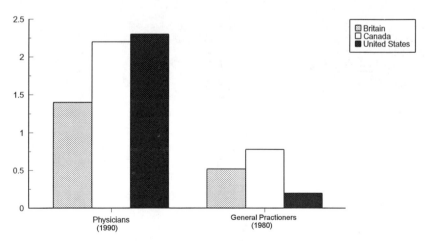

Source: *Adapted from* OECD *(1987:73),* The Economist *(1991:5).*

36 joint consultants (personal interview, NHS Executive, 1994). In the United States the ratio of GPs to specialists is 13 to 87; if one includes general internists and general pediatricians among GPs, the ratio is 34 to 66.

Governments in all three countries attempt to exercise some control over the supply and distribution of physicians. In doing so, they must contend with the power of physicians, embodied in part in professional organizations. Even though these organizations as well as their political roles are broadly similar in the three countries, governments in both Britain and Canada have had greater success than in the United States in inducing physicians to conform to national priorities.[7] Their success is facilitated by a number of factors integral to their health care systems; some of these factors involve reciprocity in government/physician relations as much as government control.

For instance, in Britain medical education is free except for room and board; in Canada tuition is small compared to that in the United States (approximately $3,000 to $5,000 [Cdn] per year). Disparities in the costs of medical education are heightened by differences in tuition across states and universities within the United States.[8] The central government in Britain and provincial governments in Canada directly control the number of places in medical schools as well as specialist slots. Britain has the strongest central government control over the employment and distribution of physicians. The Canadian provinces have failed to win the legal right to control directly the distribution and location of physician practices, but provincial governments continue to seek alternatives. Physician education and employment in the United States are competitively based and essentially market determined. Government actors in the United States attempt to offer financial inducements to both universities and medical students to reduce problems of maldistribution, but without much consequence.

In addition, both Britain and Canada indirectly employ the referral system to control utilization of health care, and therefore the supply and distribution of physicians. In both Britain and Canada GPs must refer patients to specialists. In Canada the choice of both GPs and specialists is relatively open to the patient. In principle, free choice of GPs, but not specialists, exists in Britain, but few patients exercise this right, retaining neighborhood GPs until a change of residence occurs (OECD 1992a:115). Specialists in the

United States who are not in managed-care networks do not generally depend on GPs for referrals, and in fact, specialists refer patients to each other. Although in principle there is free choice of physician in the United States, patients' economic situations and insurance determine access. Also, no matter the insurance system or country, area of residence and mobility affect actual freedom of choice.

How physicians are paid is also integral to the reciprocity/incentive mechanisms of controlling supply and distribution in all three countries. In general, payment systems in Britain and Canada not only enable direct government control but also enhance government's capacity to induce physician compliance with national priorities. Much of the temper of the relationship between physicians and government revolves around issues of remuneration—more so, however, in Canada and the United States than in Britain.

British GPs are paid on a capitation basis and work out of their own offices or in clinics; group practices are becoming increasingly common. Specialists are salaried and work in hospitals. Decisions about changes in remuneration are relegated to a quasi-nongovernmental organization, the Review Body, which considers briefs from doctors' associations, proposals from the Ministry of Health, the government's current budget plans, and data on cost of living factors. However, the newly forming, self-governing hospital trusts negotiate salaries directly with the specialists they hire. British doctors have not been as confrontational as those in the other two countries. Militancy in Britain has been greatest among other health care professionals, particularly hospital workers organized by unions.

Although physicians in Canada are paid on a fee-for-service basis by provincial governments, they consider themselves to be in private practice. Fee differences between GPs and specialists in Canada, as well as among groups of specialists, have caused much contention recently. In each province, increases in the overall fee schedule are negotiated between the medical association and the provincial government. Each provincial medical association then distributes the overall increase among the categories of physicians. Thus, the medical associations are relatively powerful in determining physician payments. Yet, of the three countries, physicians in Canada have been the most confrontational in their relations with government. Each step in the construction of Canada's Medicare program was accompanied by physician strikes, a phenomenon unknown in the other two countries.[9] Nevertheless, physicians in Canada have also engaged in a strong form of collaboration with government actors in their negotiations over fee schedules.

The comparative earnings of GPs relative to average national income is approximately 2.4 percent in Britain, 4.1 percent in Canada, and 5.1 percent in the United States. Physicians in the United States have by and large managed to ward off any incursions of "socialized" medicine; they determine their private fees on the basis of market factors. Figure 6.3 illustrates the greater earning power of specialists in the United States compared to Canada. This information implies power; it also suggests one reason for physician resistance to change in the United States. Interestingly, the introduction of diagnosis-related groups (DRGs) and the Medicare Fee Schedule, although met with verbal complaints and organized lobbying, did not engender ugly confrontations. At the same time, because physician incomes are a large part of health care expenditures in Canada and the United States (but a distant second to hospitals—see figure 6.6), these two governments have a

FIGURE 6.3   *Physician Income by Specialty*

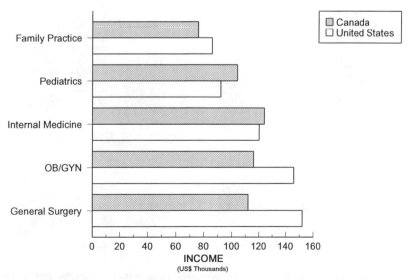

Source: Adapted from GAO (1991:39).

clear focus for cost control (Fuchs and Hahn 1990:886). Government actors in the United States and Canada have taken strong measures to control increases in physician payments.[10] Some physicians have responded by increasing the number of visits or performing more services. Some of this behavior is captured by figure 6.4, which shows the high rate of contacts per person (that is, revisits) for Canadian doctors. The data also substantiate the belief that, befitting the incentives of fee-for-service versus capitation payment, GPs in Britain work fewer hours. But they also see more patients for less time.

Each of the payment structures contains its own peculiar incentive and disincentive mechanisms. In general, salary and capitation systems encourage GPs in particular to refer more patients to specialists. Those GP groups in Britain that have adopted independent fundholding status are already showing a reversal in this tendency by treating more patients themselves. As a result, some concerns about quality control are being voiced. The fee-for-service system encourages physicians to increase the number of visits and services they provide. This behavior is more of a problem in Canada, where the overall fee structure is controlled by settlements negotiated

FIGURE 6.4 *Physician Workload*

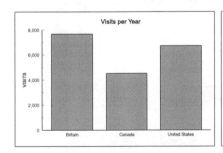
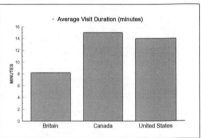
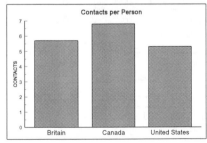
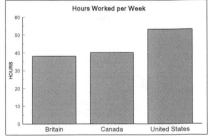

Source: Adapted from OECD (1990:46), OECD (1992:95).

between provincial governments and provincial medical associations, than in the United States, where physicians set their own fees for services provided outside of the Medicare and Medicaid programs. Whether or not the recently instituted Medicare Fee Schedule in the United States will encourage more Canadian-style "gaming" will depend in part on the extent to which it is properly implemented as procedure based rather than visit based.

One issue surrounding the dispute over incomes in the United States is the cost of malpractice insurance. Physicians or their employers are responsible for paying liability premiums, which are ten times higher than in Canada, as indicated in figure 6.5. In Canada, resort to tort law is lower in general than in the United States, and in Canada judges settle more suits than do juries, which in the United States tend to grant higher awards. Malpractice claims are increasing in Canada, but their numbers, success, and levels of awards are far lower than those in the United States. Almost all physicians in Canada belong to the Canadian Medical Protective Association, a type of insurance and counseling corporation for physicians facing legal claims. Physicians' dues to the association cover their malpractice insurance premiums.

FIGURE 6.5   *Liability Insurance*

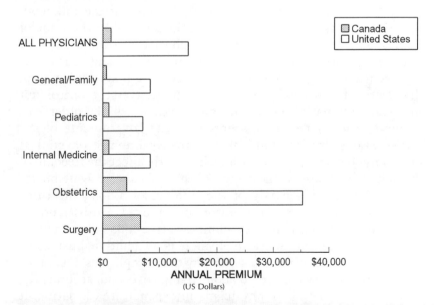

Source: Adapted from GAO (1991:41).

Litigation for medical negligence is conducted very differently in Britain. Its costs are now borne by the public sector, whose broader contribution has restrained contention in this volatile area of health care. Prior to 1990 physicians purchased their own indemnity insurance and were reimbursed in part (two-thirds) by local health authorities. Because the volume of litigation was increasing and the expense of both awards and insurance premiums rising,[11] the NHS decided to take over financial responsibility for negligence insurance for hospital consultants and specialists.[12] In a one-year transition period during 1990 the regional and district health authorities fully covered the costs of insurance and adopted the principle of vicarious liability in litigation (that is, the NHS assumes liability for negligence). When hospitals began to organize as self-governing trusts in 1991, they accepted the costs of insurance coverage for their clinical practitioners as well as all settlement costs. Hospital trusts can apply to the Department of Health for loans for unusually large settlements. Complaints about the loan arrangements led the Department of Health to institute one further change: as of 1994 an NHS central fund is being established through hospital trust contributions to handle the entire process of insurance and litigation. The Department of Health decided that the central fund arrangement was preferable to resorting to the commercial sector for insurance coverage, because of the unknown vagaries of market forces. In addition, documents on the issue of medical negligence and litigation emphasize the importance of continuing work on risk management and clinical audits as forms of prevention and control that are directly undertaken by groups of physicians themselves. The result is neither state control nor physician domination, but a mutually negotiated social order.

Few of the regulations dispensed by the governments of the United States, Britain, and Canada directly impinge on clinical autonomy; however, all regulations indirectly affect the freedom of physicians to choose the best and fullest medical care available for their patients. An anomaly of the differences among the three countries is the greater clinical autonomy enjoyed by British physicians and the greater burden of administrative constraints increasingly being placed on American physicians. In addition, businesses in the United States, insofar as they pay their employees' insurance premiums, are very concerned about rising costs and, accordingly, are examining the role of physicians in expenditure escalation. It has been estimated that in the OECD countries in general, physicians' medical decisions account for 90 percent of total health care expenditures (Immergut 1990:5).[13] This role exists regardless of the reimbursement system in any country, although not necessarily to the same extent.

As a result, a growing cost control mechanism in all the countries under study is the development of utilization and quality assurance reviews to identify physician overuse of medical resources. These efforts are most refined in the United States, where they are centered at the level of hospital care. In Canada the provinces exercise utilization review through committees with powers only to identify and notify errant physicians. Up to now physicians in Britain have exercised an extraordinary measure of clinical autonomy within the confines of the NHS budget. The government now actively encourages physicians to develop their own peer review mechanisms. Although the official rationale for medical audits is documentation of clinical judgment, all actors are aware of government's interest in resource control. Where peer review is considered insufficient, the Ministry of Health has developed direct monitoring devices, as in GP prescription rates. Overprescribers are warned but no more—yet. Despite these new developments, physicians in both Britain and Canada continue to enjoy far more clinical autonomy than those in the United States. More convergence may occur as physicians in all three countries become more involved in the processes of constructing and conducting utilization and quality reviews.

Summarizing these complexities in the role of physicians in Britain, Canada, and the United States along the state-versus-market axis yields a shallow understanding of current developments. It is more informative to note that in all three countries government and medical actors have acquired a new recognition of the inadequacies of past tendencies toward either state control or free market competition. In addition, in all three countries this recognition is melding into a new effort to develop alternative modes of decision making, as well as new criteria for evaluating health care. All three governments are playing a supportive role in these developments. Their "interventions," if they can be so called, are of a vastly different nature than in previous years. And some physicians, although far from many to be sure, are actively cooperating in the construction of new rules for an altered world of medicine.

Hospitals

Figure 6.6 demonstrates that hospital care is the largest single component of health care expenditures in Canada and the United States. Hospital care in Britain accounts for 44 percent and drugs for 10.7 percent of total health care expenditures. The mix of public and private roles makes control of hospital expenditures a prime case study for the regulation-versus-competition question. Most hospitals in Britain and Canada are publicly owned; in Canada they are governed by lay or community boards of trustees. In the United States more than 60 percent of hospital beds are privately owned, and 85 percent of these are nonprofit (OECD 1987:27–28). Data on the distribution of expenditures in hospitals reveal some important differences among the three countries, in particular the greater proportion of funds devoted to acute care in the United States.[14] As table 6.5 indicates, the United States is lowest in ratio of hospital beds per population, occupancy rates, inpatient care admission rates, and lengths of hospital stay. In terms of these categories, Canada appears to be the most hospital-oriented of the three countries. However, Canada's hospital expenditures per capi-

FIGURE 6.6 *Expenditure Distribution*

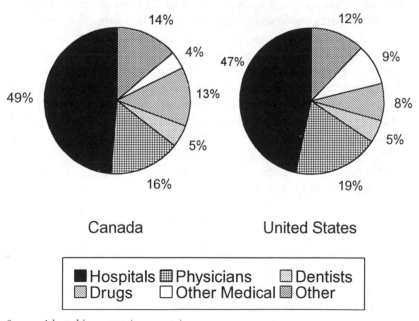

Canada   United States

■ Hospitals ▦ Physicians   ▨ Dentists
▨ Drugs   ☐ Other Medical ▦ Other

Source: Adapted from OECD (1992:23,79).

TABLE 6.5 *Hospital Care*

	INPATIENT BEDS*		OCCUPANCY RATES†	INPATIENT CARE ADMISSION RATES‡		LENGTH OF STAY (DAYS)		EMPLOYEES PER BED
	1980	1990	1986	1980	1990	1980	1990	1990
Britain	8.1	5.9	80.6%	13.6%	19.3%	19.1	14.0	2.6
Canada	6.9	6.3	85.4	14.9	14.1	13.4	13.9	2.4
United States	5.9	4.7	68.4	17.1	13.7	10.0	9.1	3.5

* Per 1,000 population.
† Percent of total beds.
‡ Per total population.

Sources: Adapted from OECD *(1987:64-66),* OECD *(1990:149),* OECD *(1992b:93-94), Schieber, Poulier, and Greenwald (1994:106-107).*

ta are 18 percent lower than those in the United States (GAO 1991:46). One reason for this is the use of global budgets for hospitals in both Canada and Britain. This single item—a macrolevel form of government control that allows for considerable, though bounded, provider decision making—constitutes a major strategy of cost containment.

In addition, both Canada and Britain separate hospital budgets for current operating costs from budgets for new facility construction and capital acquisition. This practice permits closer control of another key factor behind their lower hospitals costs: less use of technology. Table 6.6 presents data on surgery rates as an indicator of availability of technology, demonstrating the overall lower service intensity in Canadian and British hospitals for major operations. Besides (and perhaps because of) the lower rates of surgeries, studies are also finding better postoperative outcomes in Canada.[15] The GAO (1990:47) estimates that growth in the use of hospital resources accounts for only 19 percent of hospital costs in Ontario and 80 percent of those in the United States. Differences in hospital costs are also due to reduced administration in the two public systems, as noted earlier. Hospital administration costs in Canada are approximately $50 per person compared with $162 per person in the United States, according to the GAO (1991:47).

In sum, cost inefficiency occurs when the system of financing encourages greater use of hospital care. Separate budgets for inpatient, outpatient, and community care make it more difficult to reduce overall costs unless savings can be recouped; otherwise, providers spend to the allowable limits. Global budgeting, in contrast, offers providers more flexibility in where and how to cut costs. Inpatient hospital budgets are most divorced from outpatient care in the United States, especially under the DRGs. Some Canadian provinces have attempted to combine hospital, outpatient, and community care under comprehensive global budgeting, with limited success thus far. Britain has gone the furthest in consolidating comprehensive care under single hospital operating budgets, attempting to develop community care programs as less expensive adjuncts or alternatives to hospital care. Longer hospital stays are reserved for medically necessary conditions. Although government actors are central to decision making, in Britain and Canada their most visible role is also the most general (global budgeting). One would expect that microlevel decision

TABLE 6.6 *Surgeries**

	CAESAREAN SECTION[†]	HYSTER-ECTOMY	PROSTAT-ECTOMY	HEART AND HEART LUNG TRANSPLANT	TONSIL-LECTOMY MALE	FEMALE	CHOLECYST-ECTOMY MALE	FEMALE	HERNIA MALE	FEMALE	APPENDECTOMY MALE	FEMALE
Britain	10.5	229	105	7.4	186	189	48	110	214	19	165	162
Canada	19.5	573	239	6.5	483	530	170	498	414	57	186	161
United States	24.7	669	266	8.0	343	390	138	314	492	63	184	150

*Rates per 100,000 population.
[†]As percent of deliveries in hospitals and maternity clinics.

Sources: Adapted from OECD(1987:18–19) and OECD (1992b:97,99).

making would be most constrained in these two countries because of their closed financial limitations. But if we examine decisions about rationing, we see that a host of alternative factors are at work—perhaps as an unintended consequence of having to come to terms with cost containment.

Rationing

The complexity of cost containment strategies is highlighted by the issue of rationing. A few studies are beginning to appear in the literature that take the study of health care outcomes out of the "black box of expenditures" to investigate deeper traits of culture and ethics among the populace of providers and in particular recipients of health care. For example, in seeking to understand how nations decide what is an acceptable level of health care, Grogan (1992) finds that Americans focus on minimum benefits. This focus appears in schemes that ration finite resources by specifying who should receive what kind and level of health care. This tendency is "unique to America," Grogan claims (1992:214). Other countries with universal coverage (she studied Canada, Britain, and Germany) tend to limit supply through their policies for reimbursing providers and for acquisition of technology. Furthermore, in the United States the calculation of allocation primarily takes individual characteristics into account, whereas decisions about rationing in the other countries reflect institutional factors in the health delivery systems.

Only in the state of Oregon (as discussed in chapter 4) is rationing explicit; elsewhere it is implicit at best, if even acknowledged. Nevertheless, providers and recipients in both Britain and Canada realize that public-sector control over the availability of technology leads, for one, to long waiting lists, especially for elective surgeries. In Britain clinical autonomy in medical decision making dominates. The issues are more politicized in Canada, where partisan provincial governments have been known to respond to public discontent and media coverage by relaxing limits on technology control and stalling hospital closures. Opponents of national health insurance in the United States have capitalized on these news stories.

Rationing raises questions about who is making the difficult decisions about access to limited resources. In the state of Oregon all categories of political, medical, and social actors—governmental, professional, and the public—were involved in some way in the process of developing consensus on a rationing plan (Brown 1991). I turn now to the one category of actor—the public—that has been given least attention in this study.

The Public

Most assessments of the role of the citizenry in constructing and maintaining health care systems focus on public opinion surveys of satisfaction. Survey researchers, as they all note, have difficulty obtaining fully representative samples, particularly in tapping attitudes among lower-income groups. Nevertheless, there has been remarkable consistency in comparative findings on the three countries in this study. As summarized in table 6.7, Americans are much less satisfied than respondents in the other two countries and Canadians are much more satisfied with their health care systems.[16] A study by Pescosolido, Boyer, and Tsui (1985) searched for causal factors in socioeconomic background and found mixed support for models hypothesizing more disgruntlement among middle- and upper-income groups, although both tendencies appeared in Britain and, more strongly, in the United States. They also found that dissatisfaction with government performance was greater among

TABLE 6.7 *Public Opinion Regarding Health Care Systems*

	BRITAIN	CANADA	UNITED STATES
On the whole the health care system works pretty well, and only minor changes are necessary to make it better.	27%	56%	10%
There are some good things in our health care system, but fundamental changes are needed to make it work better.	52	38	60
Our health care system has so much wrong with it that we need to completely rebuild it.	17	5	29
Not sure	4	1	1

Source: Adapted from Blendon and Taylor (1989:151).

Labour Party supporters in Britain, and among both fiscal conservatives and liberals in the United States. In their study Blendon and Taylor (1989) found greater dissatisfaction in the United States among blacks, the working poor, and the disabled. They also reported that Americans were significantly less satisfied with their physicians than respondents in the other two countries. Although cultural differences must be taken into account in assessing these findings, including the culture of complaint in the three countries, we cannot disregard the general sense of inadequacies despite plenty in the United States and general social acceptance of constraints in health care provision in Britain and Canada (see also Taylor-Goodby 1983). It should also be noted that studies of American public opinion find substantial concern "with the national good and with the care of others nationwide" (Jacobs and Shapiro 1993–1994:246).

Health Care Outcomes

When all is said and done, what difference does any of this make to health care itself? Cross-national comparison of health care outcomes starkly reveals the gross inequalities and inadequacies in access in the United States. The well-publicized facts that approximately 40 million Americans are now without health insurance, that three-quarters of them are lower-income individuals, and that, in addition, a large proportion of the insured are underinsured no doubt contribute to the poor American performance on health indicators. The most common macroindicators of health care outcome—infant health, life expectancy, and death rates—as presented in tables 6.8, 6.9, and 6.10, tell us only a little about the consequences of the different types of delivery systems. Health outcome at any rate is not a clear more-or-less situation. Wellness differs among groups of people, for a variety of reasons, some of which are related to their access to other social programs. To understand more fully the reasons for the comparatively low health care outcomes in the United States despite its greater expenditures, and the reasons for the relative similarity between Britain and Canada, despite their different delivery and regulatory systems, we must recall the earlier discussion of the relationship between health care expenditures and other social expenditures. Inequality, not spending, is a key factor behind differences in health outcome. Health care outcome cannot be divorced from

TABLE 6.8 *Infant Health*

	INFANT MORTALITY RATES (%)					LOW-WEIGHT BIRTHS*		
	1950	1960	1970	1980	1990	1970	1980	1990
Britain	3.12	2.25	1.85	1.21	0.79	-	-	6.41
Canada	3.70	2.73	1.88	1.04	0.68	7.80	6.00	5.50
United States	2.92	2.60	2.00	1.26	0.91	7.94	6.84	7.05

*Percent of neonates weighing less that 2,500 grams.

Sources: Adapted from OECD *(1988:42) and* OECD *(1992b:76).*

TABLE 6.9 *Life Expectancy at Birth*

Circa:		MALES					FEMALES			
	1900	1930	1950	1980	1990	1900	1930	1950	1980	1990
Britain	48.5	58.8	66.5	71.3	73.0	52.4	62.9	71.3	77.3	78.7
Canada	45.4	56.0	63.8	69.9	73.8	48.8	59.8	69.0	76.6	81.1
United States	47.9	57.7	65.6	70.9	71.8	50.7	61.0	71.2	78.4	78.8

Sources: Adapted from OECD *(1987:37) and* PPRC *(1994:4).*

TABLE 6.10 *Age-Standardized Death Rates**

	YEAR	INFECTIOUS AND PARASITIC DISEASES (1–7)[†]	MALIGNANT NEOPLASM (8–14)[†]	DISEASES OF THE CIRCULATORY SYSTEM (25–30)[†]	DISEASES OF THE RESPIRATORY SYSTEM (31–32)[†]	DISEASES OF THE DIGESTIVE SYSTEM (33–34)[†]	INJURY AND POISONING (47–56)[†]	ALL CAUSES
Britain	1983	3.6	217.6	435.2	130.5	25.1	35.0	915.8
Canada	1984	4.3	199.1	339.6	55.3	29.4	56.0	761.8
United States	1982	8.4	193.3	407.0	53.2	32.7	62.2	842.4

*Rates per 100,000 by cause of death.
† Numbers are ICD-9 disease codes.

Source: Adapted from OECD *(1987:46-47).*

social well-being, especially poverty and its consequences, ranging from poor nutrition to violence, that stem from inadequate provision or discriminatory living conditions. In the end, health care outcome revolves around these considerations.

Conclusion

Invoking the cliché that Britain is state oriented and the United States is market oriented ignores significant forms of state and market intermeshing in recent health policy developments. Britain has undergone extensive decentralization of "the state," and its government has encouraged providers to introduce competitive methods of delivering health care. The central government remains an authoritative actor, although much less intrusive than in the past. The initial stages of reform in the NHS in the early 1990s required a large increase in health care spending in Britain. Central government actors expect that improvements in efficiency and continuing government rule over the outer parameters of the NHS budget will curb expenditures in the near future. These changes have not created any significant problems for health care itself; in fact, the average waiting time for elective surgeries has declined even though the number of people on the lists has increased.

In contrast, despite the apparent strong hand of government in the United States in some, albeit limited, areas of provision, expenditures on health care rise unabated. It is ironic that both the federal and state levels of government in the United States engage in considerable micromanagement of providers and delivery without noticeable effect on expenditures. The reason may be that the burden of regulations operate without an overarching or unifying framework for health care policy.

The presence and integrity of a unifying framework distinguishes health policy in Canada. In this regard Canada is less the "middle way" in an analysis of three models than a unique case of a negotiated order for health care. The leeway offered to provinces and providers is considerable, although perhaps not as great as currently under way in Britain. However, the unity of Canada's system remains plagued by contentions over fee-for-service reimbursement for physician services.

In all three countries integrative processes are at work. Their features are still subtle, and they exist at a broad and abstract level of analysis. The argument that I have presented here for commonality despite differences is not to be taken as imputing convergence. The similarity between Britain, Canada, and the United States is occurring not in the empirical features of their health care systems but in the evolution of their liberal welfare states.

NOTES

1. In this sense, the NHS is considered an aberration in the British welfare state because it is marked by deeper state intervention than occurs in others social policy areas. Data given later in this discussion show, however, that health care is not the highest of Britain's social expenditures. In addition, the large number of uninsured in the United States makes the American health care system an aberration in the advanced industrial world and raises questions about the status of the American welfare state.

2. Many social democracies in Western Europe are also turning to market solutions for current problems in welfare state expenditures. In doing so, they are not becoming liberal welfare states because their base of social protection remains relatively high.

3. The NHS is financed by a mixture of general taxation (79% of total expenditure), national insurance contributions (16% of total expenditure, of which employees contribute 0.95% of earnings and employers 0.8% of earnings; the self-employed pay 1.75% of their income), and charges and miscellaneous payments (5% of total expenditure) (OECD 1992a:116). At present, total expenditure in Canada is divided between provincial governments (46%), the federal government (24.6%), private insurance (27.8%), and other sources (1.6%) (OECD 1995:30).

4. A report by the Health Insurance Association of America argues that basing health expenditures on GNP exaggerates Canada's cost control capacity (cited in GAO 1991:15). In general, expanding economies spend less on health care, and economic growth in Canada in the 1970s and 1980s occurred faster than in the United States. In Japan also the healthy economy, not any particular cost containment mechanism, accounts for lower health care expenditures (Rosenthal 1992:330). Conversely, since British per capita income is lower than that in other countries, it is to be expected that Britain spends a smaller share of GNP on health care. The GAO report disagrees with this observation, arguing that health care expenditures increase faster than income in the United States and slower in Canada (1991:15–16). In addition, the report concludes that it is the single-payer system that accounts for Canada's greater cost control, because it lowers administrative costs and also "has the political incentives and ability to restrain overall health expenditures" (GAO 1991:28). The study also states that "hospital budgetary and capital controls [exercised within the universal access and single payer structure] account for 32 percent of the difference in per capita spending between Canada and the United States" (1991:42).

5. General patterns of timing and sequencing of social programs and welfare state development have been similar for Canada and the United States, per-

mitting them to be ranked as the two more liberal democratic of these three welfare states. Because social policies in Britain have been more extensive than those in the other two countries, it could be considered more social democratic; however, overall social expenditures are not as extensive in Britain as in Canada. In Britain social insurance—consisting of old age pension, unemployment insurance, and sickness insurance—was introduced in the early years of this century and expanded quickly (Flora and Heidenheimer, eds. 1981:85). The programs for social insurance that were introduced during the World War I period in Canada and the United States were minimal, consisting of lower benefits and stricter eligibility criteria for old age pension and unemployment (Orloff 1993; Banting 1987). Banting examines three periods in welfare state development: economic "take-off" (the beginnings of rapid industrial development and relatively sustained economic growth); economic "maturity" (when transition to an industrial economy is largely completed); and the introduction of welfare/social security programs. The "take-off" and "maturity" periods for Britain, Canada, and the United States are, respectively, 1780–1800 and 1850; 1890–1920 and 1950; 1840–1860 and 1910. The periods of welfare/social security program development are 1910–1950; 1920–1970; and 1930–1970. Leman (1977) compares the smoother development of the welfare state in Canada and its more pronounced "boom" periods in the United States. Expansion in the United States during the New Deal era temporarily outpaced Canadian social insurance; by the late 1950s, however, Canada's expanding health insurance and antipoverty programs for families and the elderly put that country ahead in welfare state development.

6. For a comparative analysis of the effects of social policies on poverty in the United States and Canada, see Hanratty and Blank (1992).

7. The development of the medical profession, its education, status, and culture is similar in the three countries. Britain and Canada are closer in having licensure regulated through Royal Colleges of Physicians and Surgeons, which are medical as opposed to professional organizations. In the United States, certification is conducted by the American Medical Association (AMA) and licensure is legalized by the states. On the whole, the British Medical Association (BMA) has been less political and adversarial than its two counterparts. The Canadian Medical Association (CMA) and the AMA are similar organizationally but differ politically. The AMA is a powerful lobbying organization, and although its membership has been declining in favor of specialized groupings of physicians (slightly more than 40% of physicians in the United States are currently AMA members compared with more than 70% two decades ago), its political role in Washington and in state capitals remains strong. The role of Canadian medical associations is stronger at the provincial than at the national level. Provincial medical associations have developed important negotiating relations with their provincial government counterparts; in some provinces their activities resemble those of trade union organizations. In addition to these organizational and political factors, medical journals published in any one of the countries are widely read in the other two, contributing both to a cross-pollination of ideas and to similarities in orientation and practice.

8. Within the United States the costs of public and private medical education differ substantially. The range for tuition and fees for first-year students in

1993–1994 was $13,688 to $29,440 at private medical schools. At public medical schools the range for state residents was $2,420 to $14,435, and for nonresidents it was $10,396 to $43,147 (AAMC 1994:58).

9. American doctors have had relatively little to strike over, because government sets only some of their fees and has been generous, at least until recently.

10. Between 1971 and 1985 Canadian physicians' fees decreased 18 percent, whereas those in the United States rose 22 percent (figures adjusted for inflation) (GAO 1991:5). OECD (1990:51) data demonstrate that physician incomes relative to average wages have declined in a number of countries, including in the United States after the introduction of new legislation in the 1980s. It is still too soon to estimate the consequences of the Medicare Fee Schedule in the United States.

11. In the early 1990s the cost of litigation for clinical negligence was estimated at £75 million per year in England (personal interview, Department of Health, 1994).

12. General practitioners continue to be responsible for their own coverage, as do consultants with private practices.

13. Döhler (1989:178) cites a 1980 estimate that physicians generate at least 80 percent of overall health care costs. This would mean that a large increase occurred in just one decade.

14. Insofar as public expenditure on health care in the United States is disproportionately devoted to the elderly and the Medicare program, we can expect it to be absorbed by hospital care. The largest share of Medicaid expenditures is for nursing home care, which are generally not hospitals.

15. Roos et al. (1992) focused on data on postoperative mortality among elderly patients in Manitoba and New England and found lower mortality rates in Manitoba.

16. Studies conducted within an individual country sometimes offer a different view from that in comparative reports. A British study showed a decline in satisfaction with the NHS from 1983, when 25 percent of those questioned indicated dissatisfaction, to 1987, when 39 percent reported dissatisfaction (cited in Calnan, Cant, and Gabe 1993:17). However, as Taylor-Goodby has noted: "far from reducing allegiance to the NHS, dissatisfaction appears to fuel demands for extra expenditure and attention" (quoted in OECD 1995:12). Jacobs, Shapiro, and Schulman (1993) find that throughout the 1980s Americans individually remained personally satisfied with their experiences with most aspects of the health care system—a majority of respondents consistently answered many of the questions.

Chapter Seven

Why Integrative Policy Regimes?

This study has argued that the welfare state is not being dismantled. Earlier forms of welfare state organization, based on a separation of roles and relations or on state intervention in the private sector, are giving way to new forms. But the welfare state itself continues to evolve. What we are witnessing is a change in the role of the state away from provision and toward supervision. I have sought to express the emerging form of state/society relations by means of the concept of integrative policy regime. This type of policy regime represents a coalescence of prior modes of social organization as well as new processes of social construction. Its chief characteristic is collaborative decision making, which involves all relevant actors and rejects the exercise of power to defend the status quo. The state oversees decision making and exhibits a shift away from a preference for particular outcomes toward a preference for certain types of practices within an acceptable range of outcomes. Integrative policy regimes emerge because they contain features that are more appropriate to the complexity of the contemporary social order. Earlier regimes, which I called segmented and interventionist, are based on dichotomies that no longer provide adequate frameworks for policy formulation and implementation, or for understanding changes in the welfare state. State versus market, strong state versus weak state, regulation versus competition may all have been analytically useful polarities in the early development of welfare states, but the complexities of contemporary social organization invalidate such single-dimensional views of institutional processes and forms.

This concluding chapter summarizes the future direction of welfare state transformation by exploring two alternative explanations for the kinds of changes in health policy that I have documented in this study. Both alternatives depict current developments as adaptations to the exigencies of modern society, but neither explains the continuing evolution of the welfare state. The policy regimes framework does.

One alternative explanation focuses on health care and its exceptionalism. Unlike other areas of social provision, the field of health care has witnessed revolutionary discoveries; unprecedented dilemmas have arisen because health care has become a highly technologically driven enterprise. Hence, problems ranging from the explosion of costs to moral questions about life and death create uncertainties that exist in no other social policy field. Current developments in health policy thus constitute unique adaptations to social complexities found only in this field. The other alternative explanation focuses on the welfare state itself and reiterates a theme raised in chapter 1. Many critics have argued that the welfare state has simply reached the limits of its growth. These limits include economic, bureaucratic, and democratic dimensions of social organization. In this view current changes in the welfare state represent an accession to a social reality the state can no longer control.

I reject the main thrust of both of these perspectives. I argue that health care is not unique in its consequences for welfare state developments and that the emergence of integrative policy regimes is a general phenomenon in the welfare state. I also argue that the limits-to-growth position reflects a misconception of what the welfare state is all about. These two explanations suggest either welfare state failure or a reduction in the authority of the state. I contend that adaptation in integrative policy regimes is less defensive and more proactive. I have argued throughout that the authority of the state in fact is gaining in subtle but profound ways. I recognize that several ever-present social forces may deter the emergence of integrative policy regimes (for example, the assertion of power, whether on the part of private-sector actors or the state itself in reaction to private maneuvers). As I indicate throughout this study, the dominance of status quo power relations returns decision making to segmented or interventionist policy regimes. In integrative policy regimes new sources of authority are at work, resting on the capacity of the state to foster and legitimate accommodative, cooperative, and collaborative decision making.

The Uniqueness of Health Care

Some observers argue that health care is unique among welfare state programs because it has become the most expensive social policy area, with the steepest increase in expenditures (cf. Califano 1986). OECD data do not fully support this position. Although growth in health care expenditures has been dramatic almost everywhere, in only a few countries does it consume more public expenditures than other social programs. Referring back to table 6.3 in chapter 6, we see that only in Canada are public expenditures for health care greater. In Britain public expenditures for pensions are highest. In the United States public expenditures for both pensions and education exceed those for health care. This mixed picture does not substantiate the fiscal uniqueness of health care. Nevertheless, growth in health care expenditures is highly visible and worrisome and is no doubt a driving factor in welfare state transformation.

Let us, therefore, consider other factors that might distinguish health care as a social policy area and perhaps account for its complicated expenditure picture. Take, first, the role of physicians. Previous chapters outlined the power that physicians have exercised in determining many features of health policy in all three countries, albeit in different measure. To curtail expenditures, all three governments have had to find methods of controlling physician decision making. This has been an elusive goal and has led governments to develop adaptive mechanisms for dealing with a powerful profession. But is this unique to health care? Judging from the works of scholars who specialize in the professions, it is not clear that physician/government relations truly diverge from relations between governments and other professions in other social policy areas, such as education or social work (see Larson 1977; Dingwall and Lewis, eds 1983; Freidson 1986). In these fields professional interests also demand increased expenditures, and the power of professions also intercedes in policy-making.

Professional development and the progress it has brought in medicine have led to technological innovations. The argument that technology has caused enormous increases in health care costs and in overall expenditures on health care is more substantiated. Newhouse (1993) suggests that more than 50 percent of the rise in medical costs, after inflation, is due to technological changes. Data are not available to make a proper comparison with other social policy fields. We can simply note that this cause–effect relationship may not be unique to health care either (technological development has also increased educational expenditures, for example). Nevertheless, based on the available information, one could argue that unique mechanisms are developing in the field of health care in response to the direct impact of technology on costs and in an attempt to control technology-driven expenditures. Let us look deeper into the relationship between technology and costs to identify these mechanisms.

Health care is unquestionably unique among welfare state programs in its focus on life-and-death matters. Who would not want to spend as much as is necessary to keep loved ones alive and in good health, to discover the causes of debilitating disorders and cures for them? Both the expenditures and the social costs entailed in advances in biomedical technology are very large. The complexity of issues in bioethics is sorely testing the decision-making capacity of all actors involved—governmental, medical, legal, familial, or religious (see Blank and Bonnicksen, eds 1994). At times, the new knowledge constantly being generated in health care seems to outpace our human capacity to absorb and assess its social implications.

This last argument for the uniqueness of health care brings us closer to understanding some of the reasons for the relentlessly increasing costs in health care. But it still does not clearly identify causes and effects in the relationship between technology and costs. Who is the agent? What is the policy response? And what about cost control? Why is support for some expensive technological innovations stronger than that for others? These questions can be explored through the concept of an integrative policy regime.

Integrative policy regimes develop because of the complexity of change and in order to establish processes of intermediation among various interests and values without asserting preferred outcomes in advance. Social actors, engaged in decision-making processes within integrative policy regimes, construct strategies that allow for flexible solutions in accordance with a number of social, ethical, and legal considerations. Cost reduction may or may not be among the considerations. Decision making within integrative policy regimes is decidedly different from either segmented or interventionist policy regimes, where preexisting preferences for the authority of the market, the individual, the expert, or the laws of the state shape decision-making outcomes.

The case of euthanasia demonstrates the features of an integrative policy regime. In neither Britain, Canada, nor the United States is euthanasia legal, but the practice exists in all three countries, and several court cases are testing the issue of legality. The many complicated considerations involved in decision making about euthanasia require that flexible frameworks be available for judging alternative values (see the essays in Blank and Bonnicksen 1993, part I). For example, some life-sustaining technology is very expensive, but expense alone rarely determines whether patients are kept alive. More important are the patient's likelihood of regaining consciousness and the patient's age. Yet these objective considerations may be secondary to subjective considerations. For instance, an individual's wish to die under certain circumstances may influence the decision making of family members, who may seek legal or illegal reprieve, or of a physician, who may administer treatment that does not violate the law but leads to death just the same (morphine injections to alleviate pain). In the end, decisions may be based on the principle of individual rights, the expert opinion of physicians, or an abstract principle that supersedes the wishes of the individuals involved. A particular outcome cannot be assumed in advance. But an authoritative ethic—the importance of intermediation among all relevant actors—does guide decision making. Despite different empirical outcomes, the decisions are all linked by the common processes of accommodation, cooperation, or collaboration characteristic of an integrative policy regime.

What is the agency of integration, the mechanism that oversees the decision-making processes in integrative policy regimes? Some mechanism is necessary because many actors are involved, including various bioethical groups and regulatory bodies in both the public and private sectors. And they presumably hold different positions on the development of technology, its implementation, and its contribution to rising costs. With so many participants in the decision-making process, how is a consistent response possible, so that we can say an integrative policy regime pertains?

The state is the agent of integration and intermediation. In today's welfare state system the state has begun to assume unique modes of authority. Welfare state actors in an integrative policy regime recognize that they cannot simply hand over to providers and/or recipients full responsibility for cost control or life-and-death decisions in health care in general, and regarding highly cost-intensive technologies in particular. In seeking to develop new methods of managing providers, patients, and costs, government actors are acknowledging that past methods of regulation and legislation, such as occurred under both segmented and interventionist policy regimes, are inadequate. The new methods of decision making utilize some of the successful means of the past, such as persuasion and information dissemination or knowledge production, as well as specific kinds of regulation. But they add many new actors and modalities. In an integrative policy regime, government is, as always, one among many social actors, but the one that has the most, and the most varied, resources to draw on for the construction of collaborative decision-making contexts. Policy as regulatory dictum is not typical in a full-fledged integrative policy regime. Courts and legislatures are arenas of last resort if negotiations fail, or for final approval, sanctioning the decisions reached. The role of the state more generally is to assure that these processes take place, to provide the arena for their implementation, and to oversee their integrity. As a result, the role of the state appears to be less visible than in an interventionist policy regime, but the authority of the state is not reduced. Integrative policy regimes are visibly emergent in the perplexing field of bioethics, and several actors are advocating processes of decision making similar to those expressed by the concept of an integrative policy regime (again, see Blank and Bonnicksen 1992, 1993, 1994).

In assuming their new role, state actors have had to adjust their contributions to health care production, which may give the appearance that the role of government is being reduced. But as Rettig (1994) suggests, governments have begun to make the costs of technological innovation "collective" by spreading its burden across public research budgets, private insurance companies, private medical laboratories, philanthropies, and the like. The goal of cost containment also becomes more widespread as a result. Gelijns and Rosenberg (1994) further suggest that these same actors—the many users and beneficiaries of medical research—have themselves begun to redirect technological innovation toward more cost-effective outcomes (vials of generic substances rather than large specialized machinery). Although cost control and various sorts of reductions may be the immediate goal of these adjustments, their unanticipated consequences are far more important for changes in the social relations of health care. Specifically, the authority of the state in guiding decision making is becoming more pronounced. Earlier chapters have shown that through a focus on control over costs, governments have been able to rally support for greater government control over health care in general. Put differently, government control over health care is a by-product of its asserted control over health care costs. Something similar is occurring in the focus on control over the costs of technological innovations. However, governance over the vast and complex implications of technological innovation is not exercised by government alone; its burden is spread across the many actors involved. And the state oversees the processes of decision making.

For their part, providers are willing to engage in the implicit constraints and cooperative processes fostered by integrative policy regimes because they recognize their own need for cost control and their own inability to engage fully in self-regulation. Providers may also willingly enter into integrative relationships because in some cases the consequences of medical technologies raise ethical issues outside the domain of medical decision making.

These developments, from external controls on health care to provider acquiescence, suggest yet another approach to the uniqueness of health care. For some time, scholars have argued that health care is becoming "demedicalized" (Fox 1977).[1] Demedicalization is far-ranging and its definition diffuse; its meaning for present purposes can be confined to three dimensions. First, demedicalization refers to professional changes among doctors themselves who, as a group, have become increasingly concerned with and active in nonmedical matters, such as reimbursement issues and politics. Physician conflicts of interest have received increasing attention as health care becomes more of an enterprise and less of a vocation. Second, and in a similar vein, demedicalization is indicative of a demystification in health care, as it becomes a business, a workplace, and a factor in gross domestic product. Third, demedicalization refers to changes in doctor/patient relations. In particular, studies report that some patients are increasingly demanding to be involved in decisions about their health care, questioning the authority of doctors, and introducing nonmedical factors into health care (witness the appeal of alternative forms of medicine and healing). Doctors in turn seek to involve patients when the medical choices are complex and include quality-of-life considerations.

Medicalization prevailed in both segmented and interventionist policy regimes; demedicalization creates conditions conducive to the development of integrative policy regimes. However, the difference between demedicalization, as it is commonly understood, and the parameters of integrative policy regimes is the imputation of a loss of authority by doctors in the former and the assertion of proactive authority on the part of both the state and doctors in the latter. In integrative policy regimes the authority of the state lies not in its power to impose a solution, but in its ability to guide actors toward mutually agreeable solutions. At the same time, medical authority is hardly irrelevant in an integrative policy regime, nor is the authority of the individual or the family. In an integrative policy regime, all these and other actors are involved in decision-making processes, but none dominates a priori.[2] Coherence emerges out of and as a result of the decision-making process. To repeat, the state is the agent of intermediation and integration. Its agency is always implicit and is activated only when necessary.

All these considerations indicate that health care has become too complex to govern in accordance with outdated rules. But it must be governed. The flexibility of an integrative policy regime is an adaptation, but one guided by the leadership of the state. Health care may illuminate better than other social policy areas the issues surrounding the emergence of integrative policy regimes. But the forces are inherent in contemporary society and the complexities it engenders. There is nothing unique in health care that calls for any of these responses. The assessment that a given level of expenditure or quantity of provision in a particular social policy area is too much or too little is a social-political determination. In each policy regime actors refer to different principles and norms to structure decision-making processes. The turn to flexible, integrative responses in preference to the sanctity of a traditional authority figure or institution (as in a segmented policy regime) or legalistic or technically rationalized criteria (as in an interventionist policy regime) appears to be occurring in response to complexities in other social policy areas as well.[3]

Welfare State Limits

The assertion that the welfare state has reached the limits of its growth predates current laments by certain politicians and social scientists.[4] Indeed, its reiteration has taken on a "cry wolf" quality, insofar as welfare state spending continues to increase. The notion of welfare state limits usually has two reference points. One is financial—that expenditure exceeds revenue. The other is political, constituting various normative and ideological indictments of the welfare state and its bureaucracy.

As discussed in chapter 1, common conceptions of the welfare state focus on its expansion while recognizing that no expansion is limitless. Built into the very conception of the welfare state, then, is the fact that some limits to its growth were bound to be reached. Welfare state tensions in the 1970s and 1980s seemed to confirm limits to growth expectations. The specific circumstances of the 1970s—an international economic crisis triggered by the price of oil—led to high unemployment rates and eventually unnerving budgetary deficits. Public expenditure continued to increase in some countries to compensate for the former, thereby exacerbating the latter. Conservative coalitions throughout the 1970s and 1980s resisted expenditure increases and, by implication, welfare state expansion, ostensibly in order to bring deficits under control. A close examination of expenditures shows that a slowdown in the rate of welfare state growth has in fact occurred.

However, explaining these changes in terms of the limits-to-growth perspective offers only a limited set of considerations. Growth and no-growth are complex phenomena; to focus on the state alone misses too much of both state and societal activities as well as their interrelations. For example, as previous chapters demonstrated, although current levels of state health care provision are quantitatively lower than in the past, or at least are increasing at a reduced rate of growth, overall societal provision continues at similar if not higher levels. The inclusion of nonstate actors into the sphere of production and delivery of services is qualitatively different under integrative policy regimes. It fosters the maintenance of social provision, although no prior assumption can be made about overall quantity. Some "load shedding" occurs, in which government delegates responsibility for both financing and delivery and offers minimal, if any, regulation. But it is not predominant. If it were, we would see more substantial reductions in aggregate provision. (These issues were discussed in chapters 5 and 6.) Furthermore, the limits-to-growth perspective would interpret new developments in the welfare state, including the possibility of an integrative policy regimes, as mere retreats in state activities and adjustment on the part of the state to the exigencies of the economy. And it would be inclined to emphasize those features of integrative policy regimes that curb expansion, for example, by including many opposing views in the decision-making process. Although there are efficiency-seeking tendencies in integrative policy regimes, they result from collaborative decision making; decisions about where efficiency is to be sought are not imposed beforehand.

I have argued that an integrative policy regime is neither a stagnant nor a reductionist social order. I acknowledge that this type of policy regime contains powerful centrist forces, verging toward a middling standard in decision making. But the inclusion of multiple actors does not necessarily result in an erosion to the lowest common denominator among opposing views. Decision making in integrative regimes depends on the capacity of the state to override the push and pull of private-sector power and to structure into the decision-making process principles and norms based on accommodation, cooperation, or collaboration.

The argument regarding the limits to welfare state growth draws attention to many valid points, including the necessity for some constraints in light of impending demographic developments. But the argument as a whole rests on faulty assumptions, which narrowly conceptualize the problem in the welfare state on the relationship between two variables only: state and economy. It does not completely ignore the role of "society," understood as citizens, recipients, payers, and spenders. But it interprets social participation to be secondary to the primary relationship between state and economy—social actors simply reinforce the direction already set toward equilibrium or efficiency.

In the field of health care, the role of social actors is constrained by imperfect information. In fact, this may be behind the economic disequilibrium in health care provision imputed by some scholars, because better-informed consumers facilitate the creation of more efficient markets (Barr 1992:750). The limits of the welfare state as instantiated in health care may be, then, directly related to the limits of consumer information. As citizens become more aware of the intricacies of health care provision, delivery, and financing, they come to recognize inefficiencies and distortions that misrepresent their interests—individual and collective—in health care. Inefficiency in health care means that overconsumption or underfinancing are occurring, or both. So when a better-informed public becomes aware of inefficiencies and distortions, it may actually demand more, not less expenditure, whether overall or in targeted areas. Economistic assumptions that a certain level of expenditure has become "too much," or even "crisis-provoking," rest, therefore, on weak foundations, devoid of the critical input of society.

In integrative policy regimes efforts are made to restore efficiency and equilibrate financing and consumption. These activities conjure up belt tightening all around, but this is a misleading image. Efficiency and equilibration may require that growth be rechanneled and that overall growth be continued so that rechanneling can occur. Consider again the case of rationing. In the state of Oregon, cutting certain procedures from Medicaid reimbursement has released funds for expanding insurance coverage. Some people consider this as nothing more than retrenchment, or as resignation to the fact of limits. Rationing recognizes the reality of limits, to be sure, and of limits to public-sector expenditure above all. But rationing also allows some expansion in health care provision—some of the money saved in one area is spent elsewhere. By taking limits into account, rationing forces questions that go beyond the issue of constraints imposed by limits. Rechanneling social resources is more than an accession to limits; it is also redistributive and can amount to an injunction against inequality. Ultimately, these are social-political problems that require mobilization on the part of several agents of redistribution.

We generally recognize now that the crisis of the welfare state in the 1980s not only was economic, but included various social and political factors too. With indications of fairly significant economic growth in the mid-1990s, and with the temper of electoral politics as volatile as ever, policy-makers are watching public opinion polls for assistance in formulating the terms of the present "crisis of the welfare state." They are finding that although the public remains critical of an overbearing state presence in everyday life, there remains, now as before, acceptance and even expectation of "an active government role as the last economic resort" (Shapiro and Young 1989:60; see also Cook and Barrett 1992). Despite some disenchantment with welfare spending and the expansion of entitlement it occasions, the public wants "a lot of services," not cuts; "people are receptive to more nongovernmental answers, but remain insistent that there be answers" (Ladd 1995:18–19). Thus, one could interpret any movements toward integrative policy regimes as attempts to involve citizens more directly in the workings of societal-level decisions about the redistribution of social resources, much as in the neopluralist vision presented in chapter 1. But this interpretation only partially captures the significance of an integrative policy regime. One caveat discussed earlier in this chapter is that professional and state actors remain active participants in integrative policy regimes. In addition, there is no transfer of responsibility to individuals in an integrative policy regime, as the neopluralists would prefer. Intermediation among all relevant actors and among their several differences distinguishes an integrative policy regime. And to the extent that the state oversees the processes of intermediation, its management function is more expansive than before.

Had we understood earlier that state expansion alone is not the fundamental characteristic of the welfare state, had we paid more attention to the many actors involved in multifaceted redistributive processes, had we been less prone to measuring the "achievements" of welfare state "laggards" against those of the Scandinavian social democracies, we might not now be so ready to proclaim the welfare state's demise. There are many types of welfare states; each utilizes its own mix of agents for its own preferred social outcome. What characterizes a welfare state is, above all, a commitment to redistribution of social resources to achieve an acceptable and ever-improving level of basic provision, whether the agents of provision are state or societal. Some scholars have suggested terminological revisions to capture this phenomenon. Rather than welfare state, Rein and Rainwater (1987) propose welfare society; Gould (1993) suggests welfare system; Pierson (1991) distinguishes social, economic, and state welfare.[5] These revisions support the argument I have been advancing about the changing role of the state in guiding a broader base of social provision.

One question that remains concerns persisting and aggravated inequalities in access to and levels of social provision. The multiplicity of providers—public and private—in integrative policy regimes may lead to a greater separation of clienteles. Whenever this occurs, there is an inherent problem of two- or multiple-tier services with variations in quantity and quality. Inevitably, the better-off steer toward private providers, leaving the public sector to care for the less well to do, whose care is more expensive and therefore devoid of the extras and amenities enjoyed by other classes. Overcoming these inequalities is the main challenge of integrative policy regimes, as of earlier forms of welfare state organization. Integrative processes attack the problem differently by encouraging collaboration among social actors at some level. It is possible that with its reduced burden the public sector can approximate private provision more closely, or that agents of intermediation would oversee more equity in overall provision. It is also possible, as I have warned throughout, that the forces of segmentation and/or intervention could reappear if social mobilization fails to achieve satisfactorily equitable outcomes.

In conclusion, important changes are currently under way in the health care systems of Britain, Canada, and the United States. These changes constitute a continuing evolution in their welfare states. They also signify that the welfare state is not being dismantled and its functions returned to market principles of organization. This statement may jar those immersed in the current travails of the welfare state, particularly vivid in the United States. Scholarship comprises many levels of analysis. In order to understand both present welfare state turmoil and its future forms, my study stands back from the fray and adopts a broad, historically based perspective that looks beyond immediate political conflicts. The current backlash against the welfare state in the United States should be compared to previous eras of retrenchment, none of which reversed evolution in the welfare state.

NOTES

1. There are similar kinds of deprofessionalization, or at least reactions against professional power and the assertion of alternative sources of authority, in other social policy fields.

2. Consider cases in which physicians conclude that life-prolonging equipment should be removed, but the family objects. In one case in the United States, an arbiter (in this instance, a court-appointed guardian) found another provider willing to continue life support (Bonnicksen 1993:6–8). As more cases occur, they will be settled collaboratively and with different outcomes.

3. For example, judges in divorce cases no longer assume that children should be placed with their mothers. They struggle with competing parental and child rights and wishes and conflicting "expert" assessments of competencies and needs. Judges have not always had to be mediators. Although some individual judges retain their traditional roles as authoritative decision makers, others have adopted flexible and conciliatory decision-making styles.

4. Pierson (1991:141–42) reminds us of similar complaints made in the early 1900s against social expenditures in Europe.

5. I would note, however, that the state can intervene in economic processes of reproduction and distribution of resources without necessarily establishing state welfare.

References

AAMC. 1994. *Medical Schools Admission Requirements, 1995–1996*. Washington, D.C.: Association of American Medical Colleges.

Alford, Robert R. and Roger Friedland. 1985. *Powers of Theory: Capitalism, the State, and Democracy*. New York: Cambridge University Press.

Allsop, Judy. 1984. *Health Policy and the National Health Service*. New York: Longman.

Anderson, Odin W. 1968. *The Uneasy Equilibrium: Private and Public Financing of Health Services in the United States, 1875–1965*. New Haven: College and University Press.

Andreopoulos, Spyros, ed. 1983. *National Health Insurance: Can We Learn from Canada?* Malabar, Fl.: Robert E. Krieger.

Apland, L. E. 1992. "Co-operative Health Service Delivery in Canada." In Raisa B. Deber and Gail G. Thompson, eds., *Restructuring Canada's Health Services System: How Do We Get There from Here?*, pp. 365–76. Toronto: University of Toronto Press.

Armstrong, David. (1976) "The Decline of the Medical Hegemony: A Review of Government Reports During the N.H.S." *Social Science and Medicine* 10: 157–63.

Ashford, Douglas E. 1981. *Policy and Politics in Britain: The Limits of Consensus*. Philadelphia: Temple University Press.

Baker, G. Ross. 1992. "Changing Patterns of Governance for Hospitals: Issues and Models." In Raisa B. Deber and Gail G. Thompson, eds., *Restructuring Canada's Health Services System: How Do We Get There from Here?*, pp. 195–206. Toronto: University of Toronto Press.

Banting, Keith G. 1987. *The Welfare State and Canadian Federalism*. Kingston and Montreal: McGill-Queen's University Press.

Barer, Morris L. 1988. "Regulating Physician Supply: The Evolution of British Columbia's Bill 41." *Journal of Health Politics, Policy, and Law* 13 (1): 1–25.

Barer, Morris L. and Greg L. Stoddart. 1992. "Toward Integrated Medical Resource Policies for Canada: 1. Background, Process and Perceived Problems." *Canadian Medical Association Journal* 146 (3): 347–51.

Barr, Nicholas. 1992. "Economic Theory and the Welfare State: A Survey and Interpretation." *Journal of Economic Literature* 30 (June): 741–803.

Barrow, Clyde W. 1993. *Critical Theories of the State: Marxist, Neo-Marxist, Post-Marxist*. Madison: University of Wisconsin Press.

Beer, Samuel H. 1982. *Britain Against Itself: The Political Contradictions of Collectivism*. New York: Norton.

Bégin, Monique. 1987. *Medicare: Canada's Right to Health Care*. Montreal: Optimum Publishing International.

Benjamin, A. E., Jr., and George W. Downs. 1982. "Evaluating the Health National Planning and Resources Development Act: Learning from Experience?" *Journal of Health Politics, Policy and Law* 7 (3): 707–22.

Bjorkman, James Warner. 1989. "Politicizing Medicine and Medicalizing Politics: Physician Power in the United States." In Giorgio Freddi and James Warner Bjorkman, eds., *Controlling Medical Professionals: The Comparative Politics of Health Governance*, pp. 28–73. Newbury Park, Calif.: Sage.

Blank, Robert H. and Andrea Bonnicksen, eds., 1992. *Setting Allocation Priorities/Genetic and Reproductive Technologies*. Vol. I. Emerging Issues in Biomedical Policy. New York: Columbia University Press.

——. 1993. *Debates Over Medical Authority/New Challenges in Biomedical Experimentation*. Vol. II. Emerging Issues in Biomedical Policy. New York: Columbia University Press.

——. 1994. *Medicine Unbound: The Human Body and the Limits of Medical Intervention*. New York: Columbia University Press.

Blendon, Robert J. and Humphrey Taylor. 1989. "Views on Health Care: Public Opinion in Three Nations." *Health Affairs* 8 (2): 149–57.

Blishen, Bernard. 1991. *Doctors in Canada: The Changing World of Medical Practice*. Toronto: University of Toronto Press.

Bonnicksen, Andrea. 1993. "Introduction." In Robert H. Blank and Andrea Bonnicksen, eds., *Debates Over Medical Authority/New Challenges in Biomedical Experimentation*, pp. 3–17. New York: Columbia University Press.

Bovbjerg Randall R. and Barbara Davis. 1983. "States' Responses to Federal Health Care 'Block Grants': The First Year." *Milbank Memorial Fund Quarterly* 61 (4): 523–60.

Briggs, Asa. 1961 "The Welfare State in Historical Perspective." *Archives of European Sociology* 2: 221–58.

Brown, Lawrence D. 1983. *Politics and Health Care Organization: HMOs As Federal Policy.* Washington, D.C.: The Brookings Institution.

——. 1986. "Introduction to a Decade of Transition." *Journal of Health Politics, Policy, and Law* 11 (4): 569–83.

——. 1991. "The National Politics of Oregon's Rationing Plan." *Health Affairs* 10 (2): 28–51.

——. 1994. "Implementing Health Reform: What the States Face." In John J. DiIulio Jr. and Richard P. Nathan, eds., *Making Health Reform Work: The View from the States,* pp. 143–56. Washington, D.C.: The Brookings Institution.

Brown, Michael K. 1988. "Remaking the Welfare State: A Comparative Perspective." In Michael K. Brown, ed., *Remaking the Welfare State: Retrenchment and Social Policy in America and Europe,* pp. 3–28. Philadelphia: Temple University Press.

Brown, Michael K., ed. 1988. *Remaking the Welfare State: Retrenchment and Social Policy in America and Europe.* Philadelphia: Temple University Press.

Brown, Sheila A. and Neil Ritchie. 1992. "Collaborative Arrangements in Service Delivery: The Example of Two New Brunswick Hospitals." In Raisa B. Deber and Gail G. Thompson, eds., *Restructuring Canada's Health Services System: How Do We Get There from Here?,* pp. 351–60. Toronto: University of Toronto Press.

Brush, Lisa D. 1987. "Understanding the Welfare Wars: Privatization in Britain Under Thatcher." *Berkeley Journal of Sociology* 32: 261–79.

Bunce, Valerie and Alexander Hicks. 1987. "Capitalisms, Socialisms, and Democracy." *Political Power and Social Theory* 6: 89–132.

Burgess, Michael. 1990. "Introduction: Competing Perspectives of Canadian Federalism." In Michael Burgess, ed., *Canadian Federalism: Past, Present, and Future,* pp. 1–6. Leicester: Leicester University Press.

Burney, I. and J. Paradise. 1987."Medicare Physician Participation and Assignment." *Health Affairs* 6 (Summer): 107–20.

Burwell, Brian O. and Marilyn P. Rymer. 1987. "Trends in Medicaid Eligibility: 1975 to 1985." *Health Affairs* 6 (Winter): 30–45.

Butler, John. 1992. *Patients, Policies, and Politics: Before and After Working for Patients.* Buckingham, England: Open University Press.

Buxton, Martin, Tim Packwood, and Justin Keen. 1989. *Resource Management: Process and Progress: Monitoring the Six Acute Hospital Pilot Sites.* (June). Uxbridge, England: Health Economics Research Group, Brunel University.

——. 1991. *Final Report of the Brunel University Evaluation of Resource Management*. Uxbridge, England: Health Economics Research Group, Brunel University.

Califano, Joseph A., Jr. 1986. *America's Health Care Revolution*. New York: Simon and Schuster.

Calnan, Michael, Sarah Cant, and Jonathan Gabe. 1993. *Going Private: Why People Pay for Their Health Care*. Buckingham, England: Open University Press.

Cambridge Training and Development Ltd. No date. *Medical Audit and the Manager*. Bristol, England: NHS Training Directorate.

——. No date. *Medical Audit and the Manager: Workbook*. Bristol, England: NHS Training Directorate.

Campbell, Ellen S. and Gary M. Fournier. 1993. "Certificate-of-Need Deregulation and Indigent Hospital Care." *Journal of Health Politics, Policy, and Law* 18 (4): 904–25.

Campion, Frank D. 1984. *The AMA and U.S. Health Policy Since 1940*. Chicago: Chicago Review Press.

Cawson, Alan. 1982. *Corporatism and Welfare: Social Policy and State Intervention in Britain*. London: Heinemann Educational Books.

——. 1986. *Corporatism and Political Theory*. Oxford, England: Basil Blackwell.

Central Consultants and Specialists Committee. 1989. *Resource Management Initiative: An Evaluation of the Six Experimental Sites*. London: British Medical Association.

Chandra, Jeff and Andrew Kakabadse. 1985. *Privatization and the National Health Service*. Aldershot, England: Gower.

Chirba-Martin, Mary Ann and Troyen A. Brennan. 1994. "The Critical Role of ERISA in State Health Reform." *Health Affairs* 13 (Spring): 142–56.

CLHIA. 1991. *Canadian Life and Health Insurance Facts*. Toronto: Canadian Health and Life Insurance Association.

CMA. 1992. "Ministers of Health Move Quickly to Adopt Several Recommendations from the Barer/Stoddart Report." CMA *News 1* (March 1): 2.

Contandriopoulos, André-Pierre, Claudine Laurier, and Louise-Hélène Trottier. 1986. "Toward an Improved Work Organization in the Health Services Sector: From Administrative Rationalization to Professional Rationality." In Robert G. Evans and Greg L. Stoddart, eds., *Medicare at Maturity: Achievements, Lessons and Challenges*, pp. 287–324. Calgary: The University of Calgary Press.

Cook, Fay Lomax and Edith J. Barrett. 1992. *Support for the American Welfare State: The Views of Congress and the Public*. New York: Columbia University Press.

Culyer, A. J. and Andrew Meads. 1992. "The United Kingdom: Effective,

Efficient, Equitable?" *Journal of Health Politics, Policy, and Law* 17 (4): 667–88.

Day, Patricia and Rudolf Klein. 1983. "The Mobilization of Consent Versus the Management of Conflict: Decoding the Griffiths Report." *British Medical Journal* 287 (10 December): 1813–16.

———. 1989. "The Politics of Modernization: Britain's National Health Service in the 1980s." *The Milbank Quarterly* 67 (1): 1–39.

Deber, Raisa B., John E. F. Hastings, and Gail G. Thompson. 1991. "Health Care in Canada: Current Trends and Issues." *Journal of Public Health Policy* (Spring): 72–82.

Deber, Raisa B. and S. Heiber. 1988. "Freedom, Equality, and the Charter of Rights: Regulating Physician Reimbursement." *Canadian Public* 31 (4): 566–89.

Deber, Raisa B., Gail G. Thompson, and Peggy Leatt. 1988. "Technology Acquisition in Canada." *International Journal of Technology Assessment in Health Care* 4: 185–206.

Deber, Raisa B. and Eugene Vayda. 1985. "The Environment of Health Policy Implementation: The Ontario, Canada, Example." In Walter W. Holland, Roger Detels, and George Knox, eds., *Oxford Textbook of Public Health*, pp. 441–61. Oxford: Oxford University Press.

DHSS. 1986. *Health Services Management: Resource Management (Management Budgeting) in Health Authorities.* Department of Health and Social Security, HN(86)34 (November).

DiIulio, John J., Jr., Richard P. Nathan, and Donald F. Kettl. 1994. "Administrative Principles." In John J. DiIulio Jr. and Richard P. Nathan, eds., *Making Health Reform Work: The View from the States*, pp. 12–39. Washington, D.C.: The Brookings Institution.

Dingwall, Robert and Philip Lewis, eds., 1983. *The Sociology of the Professions: Lawyers, Doctors, and Others.* London: Macmillan Press.

Dobson, Allen, Donald Moran, and Gary Young. 1992. "The Role of Federal Waivers in the Health Policy Process." *Health Affairs* 11 (4): 72–94.

Döhler, Marian. 1989. "Physicians' Professional Autonomy in the Welfare State: Endangered or Preserved?" In Giorgio Freddi and James Warner Björkman, eds., *Controlling Medical Professionals: The Comparative Politics of Health Governance*, pp. 178–97. Newbury Park, Calif.: Sage.

Dommel, Paul. 1974. *The Politics of Revenue Sharing.* Bloomington: Indiana University Press.

Douglas, Jack D. 1989. *The Myth of the Welfare State.* New Brunswick, N.J.: Transaction Publishers.

The Economist. 1991. "A Survey of Health Care." *The Economist* (July 6): 3–18.

Eddy, David M. 1990. "Clinical Decision Making: From Theory to Practice." *Journal of the American Medical Association* 263 (16): 2239–43.

Epstein, Arnold M. and David Blumenthal. 1993. "Physician Payment Reform: Past and Future." *The Milbank Quarterly* 71 (2): 193–215.

Esping-Andersen, Gösta. 1985. "Power and Distributional Regimes." *Politics and Society* 14 (3): 223–55.

———. 1989. "The Three Political Economies of the Welfare State." *Canadian Review of Sociology and Anthropology* 26 (1): 10–36.

———. 1990. *The Three Worlds of Welfare Capitalism.* Princeton: Princeton University Press.

Evans, Robert G. 1983. "Beyond the Medical Marketplace: Expenditure, Utilization, and Pricing of Insured Health Care in Canada." In Spyros Andreopoulos, ed., *National Health Insurance: Can We Learn from Canada?*, pp. 129–78. Malabar, Fla.: Robert E. Krieger.

———. 1984. *Strained Mercy: The Economics of Canadian Health Care.* Toronto: Butterworths.

Evans, Robert G., et al. 1989. "Controlling Health Care Expenditures: The Canadian Reality." *The New England Journal of Medicine* 320 (March 2): 571–77.

Evers, Adalbert. 1990. "Shifts in the Welfare Mix: Introducing a New Approach for the Study of Transformations in Welfare and Social Policy." In Adalbert Evers and Helmut Wintersberger, eds., *Shifts in the Welfare Mix: Their Impact on Work, Social Services, and Welfare Policies*, pp. 7–30. Boulder: Westview Press.

Fletcher, David R. 1990. "Council Debates: OMA Position Statement Toward a Partnership for the 1990s." *Ontario Medical Review* (June): 9–11.

———. 1990. "Perspectives on Deferring the Canada Health Act Challenge." *Ontario Medical Review* (May): 25–28.

———. 1992. "Responsible Use of Health-Care Resources." *Ontario Medical Review* (February): 1–4.

Flora, Peter. 1986. *Growth to Limits: The Western European Welfare States Since World War II.* New York: Walter de Gruyter.

Flora, Peter and Arnold J. Heidenheimer, eds. 1981. *The Development of Welfare States in Europe and America.* New Brunswick, N.J.: Transaction Books.

Forbes, William F., Jennifer A. Jackson, and Arthur S. Kraus. 1987. *Institutionalization of the Elderly in Canada.* Toronto: Butterworths.

Forsyth, Gordon. 1966. *Doctors and State Medicine: A Study of the British Health Service.* Philadelphia: J. B. Lippincott.

Fox, Daniel M. 1986. *Health Policies, Health Politics: The British and American Experience, 1911–1965.* Princeton: Princeton University Press.

Fox, Renée C. 1977. "The Medicalization and Demedicalization of American Society." *Daedalus* 106 (1):9–22.

Freidson, Eliot. 1986. *Professional Powers: A Study of the Institutionalization of Formal Knowledge.* Chicago: University of Chicago Press.

Freudenheim, Milt. 1994 "H.M.O.s That Offer Choice Are Gaining in Popularity." *The New York Times* February 7: A1, D3.

Fried, Bruce J., Raisa B. Deber, and Peggy Leatt. 1987. "Corporatization and Deprivatization of Health Services in Canada." *International Journal of Health Services* 17 (4): 567–83.

Fuchs, Victor R. and James S. Hahn. 1990. "How Does Canada Do It? A Comparison of Expenditures for Physicians' Services in the United States and Canada." *New England Journal of Medicine* 323 (September 27): 884–90.

Gamble, Paul A. W. 1992. "Hospital Resources in Metropolitan Toronto: The Reality Versus the Myth." In Raisa B. Deber and Gail G. Thompson, eds., *Restructuring Canada's Health Services System: How Do We Get There from Here?*, pp. 339–46. Toronto: University of Toronto Press.

GAO. 1991. *Canadian Health Insurance: Lessons for the United States.* Washington, D.C.: U.S. General Accounting Office.

Gelijns, Annetine and Nathan Rosenberg. 1994. "The Dynamics of Technological Change in Medicine." *Health Affairs* 13 (3): 28–46.

GHAA. 1994. *1994 National Directory of HMOs.* Washington, D.C.: GHAA.

Ginsburg, Paul B. 1989. "Physician Payment Policy in the 101st Congress." *Health Affairs* 8 (Spring): 5–20.

Ginsburg, Paul B. and Kenneth E. Thorpe. 1992. "All-Payer Rate Setting and the Competitive Strategy." *Health Affairs* 11 (2): 73–86.

Glaser, William A. 1980. "Paying the Hospital in Canada." Unpublished manuscript.

——. 1984 "Hospital Rate Regulation: American and Foreign Comparisons." *Journal of Health Politics, Policy, and Law* 8 (4): 702–31.

Glazer, Nathan. 1988. *The Limits of Social Policy.* Cambridge: Harvard University Press.

Glennerster, Howard, Manos Matsaganis, and Pat Owns. 1992. *A Foothold for Fundholding.* London: King's Fund Institute.

Gough, Ian. 1979. *The Politcal Economy of the Welfare State.* London: Macmillan.

Gould, Arthur. 1993. *Capitalist Welfare Systems: A Comparison of Japan, Britain and Sweden.* New York: Longman.

Gray, Charlotte. 1992. "Ontario Medical Schools May Be Prime Targets As Provinces Pursue Enrollment Cutbacks." *Canadian Medical Association Journal* 146 (6): 1058–61.

Gray, Gwendolyn. 1991. *Federalism and Health Policy.* Toronto: University of Toronto Press.

Griffiths, Roy. 1983. NHS Management Inquiry. London: Department of Health and Social Security.

Grogan, Colleen M. 1992. "Deciding on Access and Levels of Care: A Comparison of Canada, Britain, Germany, and the United States." *Journal of Health Politics, Policy, and Law* 17 (2): 213–32.

Gronbjerg, Kirsten A. 1987. "Patterns of Institutional Relations in the Welfare State: Public Mandates and the Nonprofit Sector." In Susan A. Ostrander, Stuart Langton, and Jon Van Til, eds., *Shifting the Debate: Public/Private Sector Relations in the Modern Welfare State*, pp. 64–80. New Brunswick, N.J.: Transaction Books.

Gutmann, Amy, ed. 1988. *Democracy and the Welfare State*. Princeton: Princeton University Press.

Haazen, Dominic S. 1992. "Redefining the Globe: Recent Changes in the Financing of British Columbia Hospitals." In Raisa B. Deber and Gail G. Thompson, eds., *Restructuring Canada's Health Services System: How Do We Get There from Here?*, pp. 73–84. Toronto: University of Toronto Press.

Habermas, Jürgen. 1976. *Legitimation Crisis*. London: Heinemannn.

Hackey, Robert B. 1993a. "Regulatory Regimes and State Cost Containment Programs." *Journal of Health Politics, Policy, and Law* 18 (2): 491–502.

——. 1993b. "New Wine in Old Bottles: Certificate of Need Enters the 1990s." *Journal of Healath Politics, Policy, and Law* 18 (4): 927–35.

Hage, Jerald and Robert A. Hanneman. 1980. "The Growth of the Welfare State in Britain, France, Germany, and Italy: A Comparison of Three Paradigms." *Comparative Social Research* 3: 45–70.

Ham, Christopher. 1982. *Health Policy in Britain: The Politics and Organisation of the National Health Service*. London: Macmillan.

——. 1991. *The New National Health Service: Organization and Management*. Oxford: Radcliffe Medical Press.

Ham, Chris and Chris Heginbotham. 1991. *Purchasing Together*. London: King's Fund Institute.

Ham, Chris and David J. Hunter. 1988. *Managing Clinical Activities in the NHS*. London: King's Fund Institute.

——. 1988. *Managing Clinical Activity in the NHS*. London: King's Fund Institute.

Hanratty, Maria J. and Rebecca M. Blank. 1992 "Down and Out in North America: Recent Trends in Poverty Rates in the United States and Canada." *Quarterly Journal of Economics*: 233–54.

Hansard. April 30, 1946. *Parliamentary Debates, House of Commons*. 5th Series, Vol. 422. London: HMSO.

Harrison, Stephen, David J. Hunter, Gordon Marnoch, and Christopher Pollitt. 1992. *Just Managing: Power and Culture in the National Health Service*. London: Macmillan.

Harrison, Stephen and Rockwell Schulz. 1989. "Clinical Autonomy in the United Kingdom and the United States: Contrasts and Convergence." In Giorgio Freddi and James Warner Björkman, eds., *Controlling Medical Professions: The Comparative Politics of Health Governance*, pp. 198–209. London: Sage Publications.

Harvey, Kathryn. 1991. "Joint Management Committee Infrastructure Established." *Ontario Medical Review* (October): 29–30.

Haywood, Stuart and Andy Alaszewsky. 1980. *Crisis in the Health Service.* London: Croom Helm.

HCIA. 1994. *The Guide to the Managed Care Industry.* Baltimore: HCIA.

Heald, David. 1988. "The United Kingdom: Privatization and its Political Context." *West European Politics* 11 (April): 31–48.

Heclo, Hugh. 1974. *Modern Social Politics in Britain and Sweden: From Relief to Income Maintenance.* New Haven: Yale University Press.

Heclo, Hugh and Aaron Wildavsky. 1974. *The Private Government of Public Money: Community and Policy Inside British Politics.* Berkeley: University of California Press.

Heiber, S. and Raisa B. Deber. 1987. "Banning Extra-Billing in Canada: Just What the Doctor Didn't Order." *Canadian Public Policy* 8 (1): 62–74.

Henderson, Georgia. 1990. "Capitation Compensation Models: A Seminar Report." *Ontario Medical Review* (January): 10–11.

Henry, Jeff. 1990, "OMA/AMA Share Common Views on Clinical Guidelines." *Ontario Medical Review* (August): 10–13.

Hicks, Alexander and Joya Misra. 1993. "Political Resources and the Growth of Welfare in Affluent Capitalist Democracies, 1960–1982." *American Journal of Sociology* 99 (3): 668–710.

Higgins, Joan. 1978. *The Poverty Business: Britain and America.* Oxford: Blackwell.

Hoffenberg, Sir Raymond. 1989. *Medical Audit: A First Report: What, Why and How.* London: The Royal College of Physicians of London.

Holahan, John, Teresa Coughlin, Leighton Ku, Debra J. Lipson, and Shruti Rajan. 1995. "Insuring the Poor Through Medicaid 1115 Waivers." *Health Affairs* 14 (1): 199–216.

Hopkins, Anthony. 1990. *Measuring the Quality of Medical Care.* London: The Royal College of Physicians of London.

Humphrey, Charlotte and Diane Barrow. 1993. *Medical Audit in Primary Care: A Collation of Evaluation Projects 1991–1993.* London: Department of Health, Royal Free Hospital School of Medicine.

Iglehart, John K. 1980. "The Federal Government as Venture Capitalist: How Does It Fare?" *Health and Society* 58 (4): 656–67.

Immergut, Ellen M. June 1990. *Health Care: The Politics of Collective Choice.* Working Paper 1990/5 Instituto Juan March de Estudios e Investigaciones.

Jacobs, Lawrence R. and Robert Y. Shapiro. 1993/94. "The Duality of Public Opinion: Personal Interests and National Interest in Health Care Reform." *Domestic Affairs* (Winter): 245–59.

Jacobs, Lawrence R., Robert Y. Shapiro, and Eli C. Schulman. 1993. "Poll Trends: Medical Care in the United States—An Update." *Public Opinion Quarterly* 57: 394–427.

Johansen, Lars Nörby. 1986. "Welfare State Regression in Scandinavia? The Development of Scandinavian Welfare States from 1970 to 1980." In Else Öyen, ed., *Comparing Welfare States and Their Futures*, pp. 129–51. Hidershot, England: Gower.

Johnson, Norman. 1987. *The Welfare State in Transition: The Theory and Practice of Welfare Pluralism*. Amherst: The University of Massachusetts Press.

Kamerman, Sheila B. 1989. "Conclusion: Continuing the Discussion and Taking a Stand." In Sheila B. Kamerman and Alfred J. Kahn, eds., *Privatization and the Welfare State*, pp. 261–70. Princeton: Princeton University Press.

Keymer, Marjorie. 1991. "Physician Resources Planning Advisory Committee (Board Agenda)." *Mimeo*. Toronto, Canada: Ontario Medical Association.

King's, Fund. 1985. *NHS Management Perspectives for Doctors*. London: King's Fund Institute.

——. 1989. *Managed Competition: A New Approach to Health Care in Britain*. London: King's Fund Institute.

Klein, Rudolf. 1983. *The Politics of the National Health Service*. New York: Longman.

——. 1984. "The Politics of Ideology vs. the Reality of Politics: The Case of Britain's National Health Service in the 1980's." *Health and Society* 62 (1): 82–109.

Klein, Rudolf and Ellie Scrivens. 1985. "The Welfare State: From Crisis to Uncertainty." *Journal of Public Policy* 5 (2): 141–53.

Korpi, Walter. 1983. *The Democratic Class Struggle*. London: Routledge and Kegan Paul.

Krasner, Stephen D. 1983. "Structural Causes and Regime Consequences: Regimes as Intervening Variables." In Stephen D. Krasner, ed., *International Regimes*, pp. 1–21. Ithaca: Cornell University Press.

Krieger, Joel. 1986. *Reagan, Thatcher, and the Politics of Decline*. Cambridge: Polity Press.

Ladd, Everett Carll. 1995. "The 1994 Congressional Elections: The Post-industrial Realignment Continues." *Political Science Quarterly* 110 (1): 1–23.

Laing and Buisson. 1988/89. *Laing's Review of Private Healthcare*. London: Laing and Buisson.

——. 1992. *Laing's Review of Private Healthcare*. London: Laing and Buisson.

——. 1993. *Laing's Review of Private Healthcare*. London: Laing and Buisson.

Langstaff, James H. 1987. "Medical Manpower: Planning/Impact Analysis." *Dimensions* (February): 31–33.

Langwell, Kathryn M. 1990. "Structure and Performance of Health Maintenance Organizations: A Review." *Health Care Financing Review* 12 (1): 71–79.

Larson, Magali Sarfatti. 1977. *The Rise of Professionalism: A Sociological Analysis.* Berkeley: University of California Press.

Leman, Christopher. 1977. "Patterns of Policy Development: Social Security in the United States and Canada." *Public Policy* 25 (2): 261–91.

——. 1980. *The Collapse of Welfare Reform: Political Institutions, Policy, and the Poor in Canada and the United States.* Cambridge: The MIT Press.

Levit, Katherine, et al. 1994. "National Health Spending Trends, 1960–1993." *Health Affairs* 3 (5): 14–31.

Lindblom, Charles E. 1977. *Politics and Markets: The World's Political-Economic Systems.* New York: Basic Books.

Linton, A. L., D. K. Peachey, and B. T. Boadway. 1990. "New Models for Physician Compensation: Caveat Emptor." *Ontario Medical Review* (February): 24–33.

Lomas, Jonathan and Morris L. Barer. 1986. "And Who Shall Represent the Public Interest? The Legacy of Canadian Health Manpower Policy." In Robert G. Evans and Greg L. Stoddart, eds., *Medicare at Maturity: Achievements, Lessons and Challenges,* pp. 221–86. Calgary: The University of Calgary Press.

Lomas, Jonathan, Catherine Fooks, Thomas Rice, and J. Roberta Labelle. 1989. "Paying Physicians in Canada: Minding Our P's and Q's." *Health Affairs* 8 (Spring): 80–102.

Luft, Harold S. 1987. *Health Maintenance Organizations.* New Brunswick, NJ: Transaction Books.

——. 1980. "Assessing the Evidence on HMO Performance." *Health and Society* 58 (4): 501–36.

Lundqvist, Lennart J. 1988. "Privatization: Towards a Concept for Comparative Analysis." *Journal of Public Opinion* 8 (1): 1–19.

MacLean, Mary Beth and Peter Mix. 1991. "Measuring Hospital Productivity and Output: The Omission of Outpatient Services." *Health Reports* 3: 229–43.

Mahler, Gregory S. 1987. *New Dimensions of Canadian Federalism: Canada in a Comparative Perspective.* Rutherford, N.J.: Fairleigh Dickinson University Press.

Marmor, Theodore R. 1973. *The Politics of Medicare.* Chicago: Aldine Publishing.

Marshall, T. H. 1950. *Citizenship and Social Class.* Cambridge: Cambridge University Press.

Martin, Ross M. 1983. "Pluralism and the New Corporatism." *Political Studies* 31: 86–102.

Mayerson, Allen L. 1968. "State Laws and Health Insurance." In *Private*

Health Insurance and Medical Care: Conference Papers, pp. 19–42. Washington, D.C.: U.S. Department of Health, Education, and Welfare.

Mendelson, Michael and Terry Sullivan. 1990. "Impediments in Reorienting Health Policy." Unpublished manuscript.

Ministry of Community and Social Services, Ministry of Health, and Ministry of Citizenship, Ontario. 1991. *Redirection of Long-Term Care and Support Services in Ontario*. Toronto: Queen's Printer for Ontario.

Ministry of Health. 1962. *A Hospital Plan for England and Wales*. Cmnd. 1604, London: HMSO.

——. 1989a. *Working for Patients*. London: HMSO.

——. 1989b. "Self-governing Hospitals," Working Paper 1. *Working for Patients*. London: HMSO.

——. 1989c. "Funding and Contracts for Hospital Services," Working Paper 2. *Working for Patients*. London: HMSO.

——. 1989d. "Practice Budgets for General Medical Practitioners," Working Paper 3. *Working for Patients*. London: HMSO.

——. 1989e. "Medical Audit," Working Paper 6. *Working for Patients*. London: HMSO.

——. 1989f. "NHS Consultants: Appointments, Contracts, and Distinction Awards," Working Paper 7. *Working for Patients*. London: HMSO.

Ministry of Health, Ontario. 1992. *Managing Health Care Resources*. Toronto: Ontario Ministry of Health.

Mishra, R. 1984. *The Welfare State in Crisis*. Brighton, England: Harvester.

Mohan, John and Kevin J. Woods. 1985 "Restructuring Health Care: The Social Geography of Public and Private Health Care Under the British Conservative Government." *International Journal of Health Services* 15 (2): 197–215.

Moon, J. Donald, ed. 1988. *Responsibility, Rights, and Welfare: The Theory of the Welfare State*. Boulder: Westview.

Morone, James A. and Andrew B. Dunham. 1985. "Slouching Toward National Health Insurance: The New Health Care Politics." *Yale Journal on Regulations* 2 (2): 263–91.

Murray, Charles. 1984. *Losing Ground: American Social Policy, 1950–1960*. New York: Basic Books.

Myles, John. 1989. *Old Age in the Welfare State: The Political Economy of Public Pensions*. Lawrence: University Press of Kansas.

Naylor, C. David. 1986. *Private Practice, Public Payment*. Kingston, Montreal: McGill-Queen's University Press.

——. 1991. "A Different View of Queues in Ontario." *Health Affairs* 19 (3): 110–28.

Newhouse, Joseph P. 1993. "An Iconoclastic View of Health Cost Containment." *Health Affairs* 12: 152–71.

NHS, Management Executive. 1990. *Working for Patients: NHS Trusts: A Working Guide*. London: HMSO.

O'Connor, James. 1973. *The Fiscal Crisis of the State*. New York: St. Martin's.

O'Higgins, Michael and Patterson Alan. 1985. "The Prospects for Public Expenditure: A Disaggregate Analysis." In Rudolf Klein and Michael O'Higgins, eds., *The Future of Welfare*, pp. 111–30. Oxford, England: Basil Blackwell.

O'Sullivan, Noel. 1988. "The Political Theory of Neo-Corporatism." In Andrew Cox and Noel O'Sullivan, eds., *The Corporate State: Corporatism and the State Tradition in Western Europe*. Aldershot, England: Edward Elgar.

——. 1988. "The Political Theory of Neo-Corporatism." In Andrew Cox and Noel O'Sullivan, eds., *The Corporate State: Corporatism and the State Tradition in Western Europe*. Aldershot, England: Edward Elgar.

OECD. 1981. *The Welfare State in Crisis*. Paris: Organization for Economic Cooperation and Development.

——. 1985. *Social Expenditure 1960–1990: Problems of Growth and Control*. Paris: Organization for Economic Cooperation and Development.

——. 1987. *Financing and Delivering Health Care: A Comparative Analysis of OECD Countries*. Paris: Organization for Economic Cooperation and Development.

——. 1988. *The Future of Social Protection*. Paris: Organization for Economic Cooperation and Development.

——. 1990. *Health Care Systems in Transition: The Search for Efficiency*. Paris: Organization for Economic Cooperation and Development.

——. 1992a. *The Reform of Health Care: A Comparative Analysis of Seven OECD Countries*. Paris: Organization for Economic Cooperation and Development.

——. 1992b. *U.S. Health Care at the Crossroads*. Paris: Organization for Economic Cooperation and Development.

——. 1995. *Internal Markets in the Making: Health Systems in Canada, Iceland and the United Kingdom*. Paris: Organization for Economic Cooperation and Development.

Offe, Claus. 1984. *Contradictions of the Welfare State*. Cambridge: MIT Press.

Oliver, Thomas R. 1993. "Analysis, Advice, and Congressional Leadership: The Physician Payment Review Commission and the Politics of Medicare." *Journal of Health Politics, Policy and Law* 18 (1): 114–74.

OMA. 1991, 1992. *Reports to Ontario Medical Association Council Meeting*. Toronto: Ontario Medical Association.

Orloff, Ann Shola. 1993. *The Politics of Pensions: A Comparative Analysis of Britain, Canada, and the United States, 1880–1940*. Madison: The University of Wisconsin Press.

Orloff, Ann Shola and Theda Skocpol. 1984. "Why Not Equal Protection? Explaining the Politics of Public Social Spending in Britain, 1900–1911, and the United States, 1880s–1920." *American Sociological Review* 49: 726–50.

Ostrander, Susan A., Stuart Langton, and Jon Van Til, ed. 1987. *Shifting the Debate: Public/Private Sector Relations in the Modern Welfare State.* New Brunswick, N.J.: Transaction Books.

Pahl, R. E. and J. T. Winkler. 1974. "The Coming Corporatism." *New Society* 30: 72–76.

Pampel, Fred C. and John B. Williamson. 1985. "Age Structure, Politics, and Cross-National Patterns of Public Pension Expenditures." *American Sociological Review* 50: 782–99.

Parry, Richard. 1986. "United Kingdom." In Peter Flora, ed., *Growth to Limits*, pp. 157–240. New York: Walter de Gruyter.

Paton, Calum. 1985. *The Policy of Resource Allocations and Its Ramifications.* London: The Nuffield Provincial Hospitals Trust.

Peachey, David K., Georgia Henderson, Darrel Weinkauf, and Jim Tsitanidis. 1992. "Can Medical Review Committees Control Overserving?" *Canadian Medical Association Journal* 146 (5): 693–94.

Pescosolido, Bernice A., Carol A. Boyer, and Wai Ying Tsui. 1985. "Medical Care in the Welfare State: A Cross-National Study of Public Evaluations." *Journal of Health and Social Behaviour* 26 (December): 276–97.

Petchey, Roland. 1993. "NHS Internal Market 1991–2: Towards a Balance Sheet." *British Medical Journal* 306 (13 March): 699–701.

Petruccelli, Elizabeth and Jeff Henry. 1991. "The Fair Distribution of Scarce Medical Resources." *Ontario Medical Review* (September): 5–8.

Pierson, Christopher. 1991. *Beyond the Welfare State? The New Political Economy of Welfare.* University Park: The Pennsylvania State University Press.

Polanyi, Karl. 1944. *The Great Transformation: The Political and Economic Origins of Our Time.* Boston: Beacon Press.

Popenoe, David. 1988. *Disturbing the Nest: Family Change and Decline in Modern Societies.* New York: Walter de Gruyter.

Powell, Walter W. 1990. "Neither Market nor Hierarchy: Network Forms of Organization." *Research in Organizational Behavior* 12: 295–336.

PPRC. 1988–1995. *Physician Payment Review Commission: Annual Report to Congress.* Washington, D.C.: Physician Payment Review Commission.

Preston, Bonnie J., 1992. Martin Ruther, David Baugh, and Roland McDevitt. "Outcomes of California's Medicaid Cost-Containment Policies, 1981–84." *Health Care Financing Review* 14 (1): 65–78.

Propper, Carol. 1989. "Working for Patients: The Implications of the NHS White Paper for the Private Sector." Unpublished manuscript.

Pulkingham, Jane. 1989. "From Public Provision to Privatization: The Crisis in Welfare Reassessed." *Sociology* 23 (August): 387–407.

Quadagno, Jill. 1982. *Aging in Early Industrial Society: Work, Family, and Social Policy in Nineteenth Century England.* New York: Academic

Press.

——. 1987. "Theories of the Welfare State." *Annual Review of Sociology* 13: 109–28.

Rachlis, Michael and Carol Kushner. 1989. *Second Opinion: What's Wrong with Canada's Health Care System and How to Fix It.* Toronto: Harper & Collins Publishers Ltd..

Radford, Teresa. 1986. "The Canada Health Act and Physician Manpower: Issues That Loomed Large." *Canadian Medical Association Journal* 134 (January): 162–67.

Ragin, Charles C. 1987. *The Comparative Method.* Berkeley: University of California Press.

Rein, Martin. 1989. "The Social Structure of Institutions: Neither Public nor Private." In Sheila B. Kamerman and Alfred J. Kahn, eds., *Privatization and the Welfare State*, pp. 49–71. Princeton: Princeton University Press.

Rein, Martin and Lee Rainwater. 1987. "From Welfare State to Welfare Society." In Gösta Esping-Anderson, Martin Rein, and Lee Rainwater, eds., *Stagnation and Renewal in Social Policy*, pp. 143–59. Armonk, N.Y.: M. E. Sharpe.

Rettig, Richard A. 1994. "Medical Innovation Duels Cost Containment." *Health Affairs* 13 (3): 7–27.

Roos, L. L., E. S. Fisher, R. Brazauskas, M. Sharp, and E. Shapiro. 1992. "Health and Surgical Outcomes in Canada and the United States." *Health Affairs* 11 (2): 56–72.

Rose, Richard. 1989. "Welfare: The Public/Private Mix." In Sheila B. Kamerman and Alfred J. Kahn, eds., *Privatization and the Welfare State*, pp. 73–95. Princeton: Princeton University Press.

Rosenthal, Marilynn M. 1992. "Systems, Strategies, and Some Patient Encounters: A Discussion of Twelve Countries." In Marilynn M. Rosenthal and Marcel Frenkel, eds., *Health Care Systems and Their Patients: An International Perspective.* Boulder: Westview Press.

Roth, Guenther and Claus Wittich, eds. 1978. *Max Weber: Economy and Society.* Vol. 1. Berkeley: University of California Press.

Royal Commission on National Health Insurance. 1926. *Report of the Royal Commision on National Health Insurance.* London: HMSO.

Ruggie, Mary. 1984. *The State and Working Women: A Comparative Study of Britain and Sweden.* Princeton: Princeton University Press.

——. 1992. "The Paradox of Liberal Intervention: Health Policy and the American Welfare State." *American Journal of Sociology* 97 (4): 919–43.

Russell, Peter A. 1990. "The Jurisdictional Pendulum Within Canadian Federalism, 1867–1980." In Michael Burgess, ed., *Canadian Federalism: Past, Present, and Future*, pp. 40–59. Leicester, England: Leicester University Press.

Schieber, George J., Jean-Pierre Poullier, and Leslie M. Greenwald. 1994. "Health System Performance in OECD Countries, 1980–1992." *Health Affairs* 13 (4): 100–12.

Schmidt, Manfred G. 1983. "The Welfare State and the Economy in the Periods of Crisis." *European Journal of Political Research* 11: 1–25.

Schulz, Rockwell and Steve Harrison. 1984. "Consensus Management in the British National Health Service: Implications for the United States?" *Health and Society* 62 (4): 657–81.

Shapiro, Robert Y. and John T. Young. 1989. "Public Opinion and the Welfare State: The United States in Comparative Perspective." *Political Science Quarterly* 104 (1): 59–89.

Simeon, Richard and Ian Robinson. 1990. *State, Society and the Development of Canadian Federalism.* Toronto: University of Toronto Press.

Skocpol, Theda. 1985. "Bringing the State Back In: Strategies of Analysis in Current Research." In Peter Evans, Dietrich Rueschemeyer, and Theda Skocpol, eds., *Bringing the State Back In*, pp. 3–37. New York: Cambridge University Press.

——. 1992. *Protecting Soldiers and Mothers: The Political Origins of Social Policy in the United States.* Cambridge: Harvard University Press.

Skocpol, Theda and Edwin Amenta. 1986. "States and Social Policies." *Annual Review of Sociology* 12: 131–57.

Skocpol, Theda and John Ikenberry. 1983. "The Political Formation of the American Welfare State in Historical and Comparative Perspective." *Comparative Social Research* 6: 87–148.

Smedley, Elaine, Jeffrey Worrall, Brenda Leese, and Roy Carr-Hill. 1989. *A Costing Analysis of General Practice Budgets.* NHS White Paper, Occasional Paper 8 (July).

Smith, Bruce L. R. and D. C. Hague, ed. 1971. *The Dilemma of Accountability in Modern Government: Independence Versus Control.* New York: Macmillan.

Smith, Steven Rathgeb and Deborah A. Stone. 1988. "The Unexpected Consequences of Privatization." In Michael K. Brown, ed., *Remaking the Welfare State: Retrenchment and Social Policy in America and Europe*, pp. 232–52. Philadelphia: Temple University Press.

Soderstrom, Lee. 1978. *The Canadian Health System.* London: Croom Helm Ltd..

Sparer, Michael S. 1993. "States and the Health Care Crisis." *Journal of Health Politics, Policy, and Law* 18 (2): 503–13.

Starr, Paul. 1982. *The Social Transformation of Medicine: The Rise of a Sovereign Profession and the Making of a Vast Industry.* New York: Basic Books.

——. 1989. "The Meaning of Privatization." In Sheila B. Kamerman and

Alfred J. Kahn, eds., *Privatization and the Welfare State*, pp. 15–48. Princeton: Princeton University Press.

Stephens, John D. 1979. *The Transition from Capitalism to Socialism.* London: Macmillan.

Stern, Morag and Sean Brennan. no date. *Medical Audit in the Hospital and Community Health Service.* London: Department of Health.

Stevens, Robert and Rosemary Stevens. 1974. *Welfare Medicine in America: A Case Study of Medicaid.* New York: The Free Press.

Stoddart, Greg L. and Morris L. Barer. 1992. "Toward Integrated Medical Resource Policies for Canada: 2. Promoting Change—General Themes." *Canadian Medical Association Journal* 146 (5): 697–712.

——. 1992. "Toward Integrated Medical Resource Policies for Canada: 3. Analytic Framework for Policy Development." *Canadian Medical Association Journal* 146 (7): 1169–74.

Stoddart, Greg L. and Roberta J. Labelle. 1985. *Privatization in the Canadian Health Care System: Assertions, Evidence, Ideology, and Options.* Ottawa: Health and Welfare Canada.

Tarman, Vera Ingrid. 1990. *Privatization and Health Care: The Case of Ontario Nursing Homes* Toronto: Garamond Press.

Taylor, Malcolm G. 197... *Health Insurance and Canadian Public Policy: The Seven Decisions That Created the Canadian Health Insurance System.* Montreal: McGill–Queen's University Press.

——. 1986. "The Canadian Health Care System, 1974–1984." In Robert G. Evans and Greg L. Stoddart, eds., *Medicare at Maturity: Achievements, Lessons, and Challenges*, pp. 3–40. Calgary: The University of Calgary Press.

——. 1990. *Insuring National Health Care: The Canadian Experience.* Chapel Hill: The University of North Carolina Press.

Taylor-Goodby, Peter. 1983. "Legitimation Deficit, Public Opinion, and the Welfare State." *Sociology* 17 (2): 165–84.

Terris, Milton. 1990. "Lessons from Canada's Health Program." *Technology Review* (February/March): 27–33.

Therborn, Göran. 1987. "Welfare State and Capitalist Markets." *Acta Sociologica* 30 (3/4): 237–54.

Thompson, David. 1987. "Coalitions and Conflict in the National Health Service: Some Implications for General Management." *Sociology of Health and Illness* 9 (2): 127–53.

Thompson, Frank J. 1986. "New Federalism and Health Care Policy: States and Old Questions." *Journal of Health Politics, Policy, and Law* 11 (4): 647–69.

Thorpe, Kenneth E. 1993. "The American States and Canada: A Comparative Analysis of Health Care Spending." *Journal of Health Politics, Policy, and Law* 18 (8): 478–89.

Titmuss, Richard M. 1963. *Essays on the "Welfare State."* London: Allen and Unwin.

——. 1968. *Commitment to Welfare.* London: Allen and Unwin.

——. 1974. *Social Policy: An Introduction.* London: Allen and Unwin.

Tuohy, Carolyn. 1986. "Conflict and Accommodation in the Canadian Health Care System." In Robert G. Evans and Greg L. Stoddart, eds., *Medicare at Maturity: Achievements, Lessons, and Challenges,* pp. 393–434. Calgary, Canada: The University of Calgary Press.

Van Loon, R. J. 1978. "From Shared Cost to Block Funding and Beyond: The Politics of Health Insurance in Canada." *Journal of Health Politics, Policy, and Law* 2 (Winter): 454–78.

Vladeck, Bruce C. 1979. "The Design of Failure: Health Policy and the Structure of Federalism." *Journal of Health Politics, Policy, and Law* 4 (3): 522–35.

——. 1980. *Unloving Care: The Nursing Home Tragedy.* New York: Basic Books.

——. 1995. "Medicaid 1115 Waivers: Progress Through Partnership." *Health Affairs* 14 (1): 217–20.

Wahn, Michael. 1992. "Controlling Overservicing by Physicians: Review of Office Practices in Manitoba." *Canadian Medical Association Journal* 146 (5): 723–28.

Wallack, Stanley S. 1991. "Managed Care: Practice, Pitfalls, and Potential." *Health Care Financing Review* (Annual Supplement): 27–34.

Wedderburn, Dorothy. 1965. "Facts and Theories of the Welfare State." *The Socialist Register,* pp. 127–46

Weller, Geoffrey R. and Pranlal Manga. 1983. "The Push for Reprivatization of Health Care Services in Canada, Britain, and the United States." *Journal of Health Politics, Policy, and Law* 8 (3): 495–518.

Wennberg, John and A. Gittelsohn. 1973. "Small Area Variations in Health Care Delivery." *Science* 182 (December 14): 1102–1108.

Wilensky, Harold L. 1975. *The Welfare State and Equality: Structural and Ideological Roots of Public Expenditures.* Berkeley: University of California Press.

Williamson, Peter J. 1985. *The Varieties of Corporatism: A Conceptual Discussion.* New York: Cambridge University Press.

Winkler, J. T. 1976. "Corporatism." *Archives of European Sociology* 17 (1): 100–36.

Woolf, Steven H. 1990. "Practice Guidelines: A New Reality in Medicine." *Archives of Internal Medicine* 150 (September): 1811–18.

Working Group of the Regional Medical Audit Coordinators' Committee and Conference of Colleges' Audit Working Group. February 1993. *Audit and the Purchaser/Provider Interaction.* EL(93) Annex B. Leeds, England: NHS Executive.

Index